I0103938

# SPARK©

## A Compassionate and Informative Guide to Alzheimer's and Dementia Care for Families and Caregivers

———— ✦ ————

*Education & All The Tools You Need When Caring From the Heart.*
*Neurocognitive Exercise Games Included — Fitness For the Brain!*

Author
Lisa A. Greenlee
Geriatric Nurse Care Manager · Certified Dementia Practitioner
Cognitive Health Program Consultant

SPARK© A Compassionate and Informative Guide to Alzheimer's and Dementia Care for Families and Caregivers is proprietary, and the educational material within this book constitutes knowledge obtained in the field of nursing over twenty-eight years.

Select educational content has been referenced and used under fair use for educational purposes; all sources are fully cited and acknowledged within the text. The product of the author's shared knowledge and opinion and its resemblance to other reference material is entirely coincidental.

No part of this book may be reproduced in any form, by electronic or mechanical means, including information storage and retrieval systems, without permission in writing from the copyright owner, except by a reviewer who may quote brief passages in a review.

Copyright © 2025 by Lisa A. Greenlee
All rights reserved.

Published by WrenPen, LLC
Circleville, Ohio

ISBN: 979-8-218-73623-1

Cover Art by: Rehmat Ullah
https://www.fiverr.com/zeein2016

Library of Congress Control Number: 2025914705

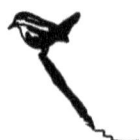

## A Message From the Author

I would like to wish you the best of luck as you embark on this journey of learning and caregiving. Supporting a loved one with Alzheimer's or Dementia is a challenge, but it also presents an opportunity to make a meaningful difference in their life. This book is designed to provide you with practical strategies, insights, and resources to help you navigate the complexities of caregiving with confidence and compassion. Remember to be patient with yourself and your loved one, and know that every small effort you make contributes to their well-being and quality of life.

Caring for someone with Alzheimer's or Dementia requires dedication, adaptability, and self-care. By implementing structured routines, effective communication techniques, and safety measures, you can create a nurturing environment that promotes comfort and security. At the same time, don't forget to prioritize your well-being by seeking support, taking breaks, and maintaining emotional resilience, which are essential aspects of being an effective caregiver. With knowledge, patience, and a compassionate heart, you can provide the best care possible while ensuring that you, too, remain strong and supported throughout this journey.

Thank you so much for purchasing this workbook and for your unwavering dedication to improving the lives of those with Alzheimer's and Dementia. Your commitment to providing the care and support these individuals need is invaluable. Together, as a team, we have the power to make a profound impact on their quality of life, helping them navigate the challenges of the disease with dignity and compassion. Your efforts are sincerely appreciated, and through this combined journey, we can empower patients to live well throughout their disease process.

# Acknowledgments

This book is rooted in years of practical experience supporting individuals and families affected by cognitive decline. I am grateful to the many clients and caregivers who allowed me to walk alongside them in the most vulnerable seasons of their lives. Your strength, patience, and honesty have shaped the heart of this resource.

I also wish to thank the interdisciplinary professionals I've had the privilege to work alongside, especially my colleagues in memory care, nursing, therapy services, and case management.

A special thank you to the many geriatricians, family practice physicians, neurologists, and memory care specialists for your unwavering dedication, clinical insight, and compassionate guidance in supporting individuals and families navigating the complexities of cognitive decline.

All material has been developed, reviewed, adapted, and guided by my professional expertise as a nurse care manager and certified dementia practitioner. Note: AI assistance was used in the editing, and organizational development of select text using ChatGPT by OpenAI. Final content reflects the author's original composition, expertise, and editorial judgment.

Thank you to Rehmat Ullah for the exceptional care when creating the wonderfully dynamic cover art.

Thank you to my family for always supporting my endeavors, no matter how big or small.

## *Still Here*

*"I see the glimmer in your eyes,*
*The spark that lingers, faint but true.*

*Names and faces may come and go,*
*But the heart remembers all we know.*

*Your hands, etched deep with time's design,*
*still echo every curve of mine.*

*Together, we will brave the fog,*
*In this most uncharted land.*

*Where memory fades like light*
*We'll walk this journey hand in hand."*

*Original poem by*
*Lisa A. Greenlee*

For My Beloved Parents & Grandparents
*Richard Allen & Monna Kay Peters Greenlee*
*Denver Willian & Helen Wren Boone Greenlee*
*Roy Mason & Prudis Conley Peters*

# TABLE OF CONTENTS

# CHAPTER 1

# Understanding Alzheimer's and Dementia

Alzheimer's disease and dementia are terms often used interchangeably, but they are not the same. **Dementia** is an umbrella term for a decline in cognitive function that interferes with daily life, and **Alzheimer's disease** is the most common form of dementia, accounting for up to 70% of all dementia cases. These conditions primarily affect older adults but are not a normal part of the aging process.

## A Better Understanding — What Is Dementia?

Dementia is not one specific disease; it's a general term used to describe a set of symptoms that affect memory, thinking, communication, judgment, and daily functioning. These changes are significant enough to interfere with a person's ability to live independently.

The reason dementia is often called an *umbrella disease* is that it covers a wide range of specific medical conditions that fall beneath it, each with different causes, progression patterns, and treatments. Imagine "dementia" as the canopy of an umbrella, and under that canopy are many different types, including:

- **Alzheimer's disease** – the most common type, known for gradual memory loss and confusion.

- **Vascular dementia** is caused by reduced blood flow to the brain, often after strokes or small vessel disease.

- **Lewy body dementia** is marked by visual hallucinations, movement changes, and fluctuating alertness.

- **Frontotemporal dementia** often begins with changes in personality, judgment, or language, rather than with memory loss.

- **Mixed dementia** – a combination of two or more types, such as Alzheimer's and vascular dementia.

Each of these has distinct characteristics, but they all share a common thread: progressive cognitive decline that affects daily life.

It's important to remember that dementia is not a normal part of aging. While aging increases risk, dementia is caused by damage to brain cells, not just "getting older." And because it affects more than just memory, care must address the *whole person*: emotional health, communication, safety, dignity, and connection.

Understanding dementia as an umbrella helps caregivers and families grasp the diversity within the diagnosis. It also encourages more personalized care, because no two people with dementia are precisely alike, and their journeys will be as unique as their lives have been.

## Disease Processes: What Happens in the Brain?

Alzheimer's disease and other dementias are characterized by progressive damage to brain cells and their connections. This damage begins years, sometimes decades, before noticeable symptoms appear. In Alzheimer's disease, two abnormal protein accumulations are central to its pathology:

### 1. Amyloid Plaques

These are sticky clumps of beta-amyloid protein that collect between nerve cells (neurons), disrupting cell communication. Over time, the immune system responds with inflammation, contributing further to cell damage (Selkoe & Hardy, 2016).

### 2. Neurofibrillary Tangles

Inside the neurons, a protein called tau becomes abnormally twisted and tangled. These tau tangles interfere with the transport of nutrients and other essential materials within the cell, ultimately leading to cell death (Iqbal et al., 2010).

As neurons die, the brain shrinks. This shrinkage, or cortical atrophy, is particularly prominent in the hippocampus, a region essential for memory formation. The damage spreads gradually, affecting different brain regions responsible for reasoning, behavior, language, and ultimately, basic bodily functions such as swallowing and breathing.

In vascular dementia, reduced blood flow, resulting from a stroke or chronic damage to blood vessels, deprives brain cells of oxygen and nutrients. Other types of dementia, like Lewy body dementia or frontotemporal dementia, involve different types of abnormal protein build-up and patterns of cell death.

Importantly, Alzheimer's is a neurodegenerative disease, meaning it gets worse over time as more and more neurons are damaged or lost. The exact cause is likely a combination of genetic, environmental, and lifestyle factors.

## Symptoms:

The symptoms of dementia and Alzheimer's disease vary depending on the cause and stage of the condition, but generally include:

**Cognitive symptoms**:

- Memory loss, especially of recent events

- Difficulty finding words

- Difficulty with decision-making

- Difficulty with planning and organizing

- Confusion about time and place

- Difficulty with visual-spatial relationships

**Behavioral and psychological symptoms:**

- Mood changes, such as depression, anxiety, or irritability

- Withdrawal from social activities

- Sleep disturbances

- Personality changes

- Hallucinations or delusions (in later stages)

## Diagnosis

Early diagnosis is crucial to managing symptoms and planning care. There is no single test for Alzheimer's or dementia, so doctors typically use a combination of the following:

- **Medical history and physical examination**

- **Cognitive and neuropsychological tests** (e.g., Mini-Mental State Examination)

- **Brain imaging** (MRI, CT, or PET scans) to detect brain shrinkage or abnormalities

- **Blood tests** to rule out other causes of symptoms, such as vitamin deficiencies or thyroid problems

- **Neurological exams** to assess balance, reflexes, and sensory function

In recent years, biomarkers—such as levels of beta-amyloid and tau proteins in cerebrospinal fluid—have improved diagnostic accuracy, especially in research settings.

## Stages of Alzheimer's Disease

*Alzheimer's disease progresses gradually and is typically divided into three main stages:*

1. **Early-stage (Mild):**

    - Minor memory lapses, especially forgetting recent events or conversations

- Difficulty with problem-solving or complex tasks

- Still able to live independently with some support

2. **Middle-stage (Moderate):**

- Increased memory loss and confusion

- Difficulty recognizing family or friends

- Trouble with language and thought processing

- Behavioral and mood changes, including suspicion and frustration

- Needs help with daily activities like dressing and eating

3. **Late-stage (Severe):**

- Loss of ability to communicate clearly

- Difficulty swallowing and controlling bodily functions

- Significant personality changes

- Requires full-time care

## Treatment and Management

There is currently no cure for Alzheimer's or most forms of dementia, but treatments can help manage symptoms and improve quality of life.

**Medications:**

- **Cholinesterase inhibitors** (such as donepezil, rivastigmine, and galantamine) help improve memory and thinking in the early to moderate stages of Alzheimer's disease.

- **Memantine** helps regulate glutamate and is typically prescribed for individuals in the moderate to severe stages of the disease.

- In some cases, **antidepressants, antipsychotics, or sleep aids** are prescribed to manage behavioral symptoms.

Recent breakthroughs in Alzheimer's treatment—like the development of infusion therapies that target amyloid plaques—mark a hopeful shift toward slowing disease progression rather than just managing symptoms. These advancements underscore the crucial role of ongoing research and development in discovering new pathways, enhancing the quality of life, and advancing us closer to a cure.

Leqembi (lecanemab) is a relatively new intravenous infusion therapy approved for the treatment of early-stage Alzheimer's disease. Developed by Eisai and Biogen, it is designed for patients with mild cognitive impairment or mild dementia, confirmed to have amyloid beta plaques in the brain—a hallmark of Alzheimer's. Leqembi is a monoclonal antibody that targets and clears these amyloid plaques, aiming to slow cognitive and functional decline. Clinical trials, notably the Phase 3 Clarity AD study, demonstrated that Leqembi reduced clinical decline by approximately 27% over 18 months compared to a placebo, resulting in a delay in disease progression of roughly 5.3 months.

Initially, Leqembi required biweekly intravenous infusions. However, in January 2025, the FDA approved a maintenance dosing regimen of once every four weeks after the initial 18 months of treatment, potentially easing the treatment burden for patients and caregivers. Despite its promise, Leqembi is not without risks. Some patients may experience amyloid-related imaging abnormalities (ARIA), such as brain swelling or microhemorrhages, which necessitate careful monitoring through regular MRI scans. Additionally, access to Leqembi has been challenging due to factors like limited infusion center availability, the need for specialized neurological care, and the requirement for early diagnosis. Nonetheless, Leqembi represents a significant advancement in Alzheimer's therapeutics, offering hope for slowing disease progression in its early stages.

**Non-drug therapies:**

- **Cognitive stimulation therapy** and structured activities can help maintain mental function and cognitive abilities.

- **Occupational therapy** to support independence in daily tasks

- **Routine and environment modifications** to reduce confusion and agitation

**Supportive care:**

- **Caregiver support** and education are essential, as the condition progresses

- **Palliative and hospice care** are often considered in the final stages to ease pain symptoms and provide comfort.

# Food for thought — Is Alzheimer's Disease Type III Diabetes?

Over the past two decades, an intriguing and potentially groundbreaking hypothesis has emerged in neuroscience and endocrinology: Alzheimer's disease may be a form of diabetes that selectively affects the brain. This theory, often referred to as "Type III diabetes," proposes that insulin resistance and impaired insulin signaling in the brain are central to the development and progression of Alzheimer's disease (AD). But how strong is the evidence for this claim? What mechanisms support this link? And what implications does this have for treatment and prevention?

# Understanding the Basics: Insulin and the Brain

Traditionally, insulin is known for its critical role in regulating glucose metabolism in the body, particularly

in tissues such as the liver, muscle, and adipose tissue. However, the brain, once thought to be insulin-independent, is now recognized to rely on insulin for several important functions. Insulin receptors are widely distributed throughout the brain, particularly in regions associated with memory and learning, including the hippocampus and cerebral cortex.

In the brain, insulin plays a crucial role in modulating synaptic plasticity, promoting neuronal survival, regulating neurotransmitter release, and enhancing memory formation. It is also crucial in maintaining metabolic homeostasis by affecting glucose uptake and utilization in neurons and glial cells. Disruption in insulin signaling, therefore, can have serious consequences for cognitive health.

## The Insulin Resistance Connection

Type 2 diabetes mellitus (T2DM) is characterized by peripheral insulin resistance — a condition in which cells fail to respond properly to insulin. Epidemiological studies have shown that individuals with T2DM are at a significantly higher risk (up to 50-100% increased risk) of developing Alzheimer's disease compared to those without diabetes (Ott et al., 1999; Cheng et al., 2012).

Research into the brains of Alzheimer's patients has found evidence of insulin resistance independent of peripheral diabetes. Studies by de la Monte and Wands (2008) demonstrated that insulin signaling is impaired in the brains of individuals with AD, and insulin receptor expression is decreased. These findings led to the coining of the term "Type III diabetes" to describe the selective resistance to insulin in the brain that contributes to Alzheimer's pathology.

## Molecular Mechanisms Linking Diabetes and Alzheimer's

There are several molecular mechanisms that help bridge the understanding between diabetes and Alzheimer's disease:

1. **Insulin and Amyloid-β Accumulation**: Insulin-degrading enzyme (IDE) breaks down both insulin and amyloid-β, the latter being a key pathological hallmark of AD. In states of insulin resistance, IDE is overwhelmed, leading to the accumulation of amyloid-β plaques (Farris et al., 2003).

2. **Tau Phosphorylation**: Insulin signaling helps regulate tau phosphorylation through pathways such as the PI3K/Akt and GSK-3β pathways. Impaired insulin signaling increases GSK-3β activity, which promotes hyperphosphorylation of tau protein and neurofibrillary tangle formation, another hallmark of Alzheimer's (Griffin et al., 2005).

3. **Neuroinflammation and Oxidative Stress**: Chronic insulin resistance and hyperglycemia contribute to increased production of pro-inflammatory cytokines and reactive oxygen species in the brain, exacerbating neurodegeneration.

4. **Mitochondrial Dysfunction**: Insulin plays a role in mitochondrial biogenesis and function. Impaired insulin signaling in neurons leads to reduced energy production and increased susceptibility to cellular damage.

## Clinical Implications and Potential Treatments

If Alzheimer's is indeed a form of brain-specific diabetes, this opens the door to new diagnostic and therapeutic strategies. Intranasal insulin, which bypasses the blood-brain barrier, has been shown in some studies to improve memory and cognitive function in patients with mild cognitive impairment and early Alzheimer's (Craft et al., 2012). Other therapeutic avenues include the use of insulin-sensitizing agents, such as metformin, GLP-1 receptor agonists, and lifestyle interventions aimed at enhancing insulin sensitivity.

Preventive strategies focusing on metabolic health — including a balanced diet, regular exercise, and maintaining a healthy weight — are increasingly viewed as vital in reducing the risk of cognitive decline. The Mediterranean and DASH diets, both associated with improved insulin sensitivity and reduced inflammation, have also been linked to lower rates of Alzheimer's disease.

## The Debate and Future Directions

Despite the compelling evidence, not all researchers agree with labeling Alzheimer's disease as "Type III diabetes." Critics argue that while insulin resistance may be a contributing factor, it is unlikely to be the sole cause of such a complex and multifactorial disease. Genetic factors, particularly the APOE4 allele, environmental exposures, and other comorbidities, also play significant roles.

Nonetheless, the Type III diabetes hypothesis has re-energized research into Alzheimer's, providing a fresh lens through which to view disease mechanisms and treatment. It underscores the importance of viewing neurodegeneration not just as a disorder of the brain, but as a systemic illness with deep roots in metabolic dysfunction.

## Preventative Measures

We may not be able to do anything about the genetic component of Alzheimer's and Dementia, but education and early lifestyle modifications are in our control. Limiting exposure to potential environmental concerns and maintaining a healthy lifestyle with a proper diet and routine exercise may help reduce the likelihood of neurocognitive decline.

## Conclusion

While Alzheimer's disease is not officially classified as a form of diabetes, the term "Type III diabetes" effectively highlights the growing recognition of insulin resistance as a central player in neurodegeneration. Continued research is needed to fully elucidate the link and determine whether targeting insulin pathways can alter the trajectory of Alzheimer's. If this connection is confirmed, it would represent a paradigm shift, suggesting that brain health is inextricably tied to metabolic health..

# CHAPTER 2

# Quality of Life as the Cornerstone of Dementia Care

When a person is diagnosed with Alzheimer's or another form of dementia, the focus of care often shifts to medical management and long-term planning. While these are important, they must not overshadow the central goal: preserving and enhancing the individual's quality of life. Quality of life encompasses more than just physical health; it includes emotional well-being, connection to others, engagement in meaningful activities, and the ability to experience dignity and joy, even as cognitive abilities change.

Alzheimer's and dementia gradually erode memory, comprehension, and independence, but these conditions do not strip a person of their humanity. Each individual, regardless of disease progression, continues to feel emotions, experience relationships, and benefit from comfort and familiarity. Prioritizing quality of life means recognizing the person behind the diagnosis, honoring their preferences, values, and history. It's not about what is lost, but about nurturing what remains.

A *person-centered approach* to dementia care fosters autonomy and inclusion, which can be achieved by involving the person in daily decisions, tailoring routines to their rhythms, and creating environments that feel safe and reassuring.

Thoughtful stimulation, through music, sensory engagement, art, nature, and conversation, can spark memory, relieve agitation, and restore a sense of identity. These moments, while often small, accumulate into a life of meaning and connection.

Families and caregivers also benefit when quality of life becomes the focus. Rather than measuring success solely by medical stability or task completion, caregivers are encouraged to measure success by moments of peace, laughter, or recognition. This reframing reduces caregiver burnout and helps sustain compassionate care through the most challenging phases of the disease. It reminds everyone involved that the goal is not to "fix" the person, but to walk with them with kindness and understanding.

Ultimately, quality of life is not a luxury; it is a right. It is the heartbeat of ethical, respectful, and effective dementia care. Whether a person is in the early stages of memory loss or nearing the end of life, their experience matters. Furthermore, when we commit to preserving dignity, honoring individuality, and fostering joy, we embody what it truly means to care.

This book was created with the caregiver in mind because they hold a sacred power—the ability to transform the everyday into something deeply meaningful. Through patience, presence, and love, a caregiver can affirm the worth of their loved one in ways that words cannot always express.

Simple acts like brushing hair gently, sharing a favorite song, reminiscing over old photos, or offering a warm hand to hold can make all the difference. These quiet gestures speak volumes: *You are still here. You still matter.*

When a caregiver sees beyond the disease and connects with the person within, they make life valuable and precious again. In this way, caregivers don't just provide care, they become vessels of dignity, preserving the essence of a person whose world may be fading, but whose spirit still longs to be seen.

# CHAPTER 3

# The Power of Presence — Why Enrichment, Socialization, and Engagement Matter

It's easy to focus on what's fading when caring for someone with Alzheimer's or dementia. Names slip away. Time blurs. Familiar routines unravel. But beneath all of that, something essential remains: the human need for connection, purpose, and joy.

Enrichment and engagement are not luxuries in dementia care—they are lifelines. They awaken the parts of the soul that still respond to beauty, touch, rhythm, and kindness. Even as memory fragments, the emotional core of a person often remains deeply alive.

We often prioritize safety, hygiene, medication, and meals, and rightly so. Physical care is critical. But without emotional, spiritual, and cognitive nourishment, care becomes incomplete. Enrichment and socialization are just as important as physical care and safety because they honor the *whole person*, not just the diagnosis. We are not merely tending to bodies—we are holding stories, identities, and relationships that still matter.

Think of enrichment as an offering—a way of inviting the person back into the world through what feels comforting and familiar. A warm cup of tea is served with ceremony. A favorite song hummed softly in the afternoon. A textured fabric placed in uncertain hands. These small moments are not idle pastimes. They are bridges. And they remind the person, even without words, that they are still part of something meaningful.

Socialization matters just as much. Dementia can isolate people, even in the presence of others. But gentle, intentional interaction breaks through the fog. It might be a smile held a few seconds longer. A story told, even if it's forgotten. A quiet presence that doesn't demand understanding, but offers a sense of belonging. In these interactions, the caregiver becomes a mirror, reflecting back dignity, personhood, and worth.

When people are engaged—when they are invited to be, rather than just being cared for—something shifts. Restlessness softens. Agitation quiets. Sometimes, even the gaze clears for a moment, and the person looks right through the disease and into you. Those moments don't need to be long. They just need to be real.

Engagement doesn't have to be elaborate. Folding laundry together. Listening to wind chimes. Holding a hand through the rhythm of breath. These are holy exchanges. And while they may not restore memory, they preserve meaning.

Ultimately, this work is about more than just managing symptoms. It's about honoring the human spirit. Enrichment and connection remind the person—and the caregiver—that life still pulses here. And where there is life, there is still room for joy.

# CHAPTER 4

# What is Neurocognitive Therapy?

Neurocognitive Stimulation Therapy (NCT) is a therapeutic approach designed to enhance or maintain cognitive functions, including memory, attention, problem-solving, and executive functioning. It primarily targets individuals who experience cognitive decline, often due to aging, neurodegenerative diseases (such as Alzheimer's or Parkinson's), brain injuries, or other cognitive impairments.

The goal of neurocognitive stimulation therapy is to slow or mitigate the effects of cognitive decline, thereby improving the individual's ability to perform daily tasks and maintain independence.

## Key Aspects of Neurocognitive Therapy:

**Cognitive Exercises**: These structured activities aim to challenge and stimulate various cognitive functions, including memory, attention, and reasoning. Examples include puzzles, word games, math, word problems, and memory recall exercises. These exercises can be tailored to a person's specific cognitive needs and difficulties.

**Brain Training**: NCT often involves exercises that require concentration and mental effort, encouraging the brain to form new neural connections. This process, known as neuroplasticity, enables the brain to adapt and compensate for areas of cognitive decline. The brain is not a muscle, but it must be treated like one.

**Repetition and Consistency**: Repeated engagement in these exercises helps reinforce cognitive skills and may prevent further deterioration. The consistent practice of cognitive tasks helps strengthen neural pathways and maintain brain function over time.

**Therapeutic Environment**: Neurocognitive stimulation often occurs in a supportive, structured environment, which may be located in a clinic, at home with a caregiver, or in group settings. It focuses not just on the individual's cognitive skills but also on their emotional well-being, reducing feelings of frustration and helplessness.

**Personalized Approach**: Therapists typically tailor neurocognitive stimulation to an individual's specific challenges, considering their cognitive assessment and particular needs. For example, someone with a memory impairment might focus more on exercises aimed at memory recall, while another individual may focus on attention and concentration training.

**Reminiscence Therapy**: This type of exercise involves sensory cues and discussions to evoke memories, making it a beneficial non-pharmacological intervention.

Keeping the mind stimulated and the heart happy is one of the most meaningful ways we can nurture ourselves and our loved ones, especially in the face of memory loss. Whether it's through music, conversation, laughter, or simple shared moments, these small joys awaken something deep within us. Staying mentally and emotionally engaged doesn't just preserve memories; it reminds us of who we are and what still matters. Even in the quietest seasons, connection and curiosity can light the way forward

# Benefits of Neurocognitive Therapy

**Improves Cognitive Function**: Helps individuals maintain or enhance their cognitive abilities, including memory, attention, and executive functions like decision-making.

**Delays Cognitive Decline**: In people with neurodegenerative diseases like Alzheimer's, NCT can slow down the rate of cognitive decline and prolong functional independence.

**Enhances Quality of Life**: By improving cognitive skills, individuals can experience greater autonomy, which boosts their confidence and overall well-being.

**Emotional Support**: NCT can help reduce anxiety, depression, and frustration by providing individuals with strategies to manage cognitive challenges better.

**Support for Caregivers**: It also provides strategies for family members and caregivers, teaching them how to assist their loved ones better and manage caregiving responsibilities.

## Who Benefits from Neurocognitive Therapy?

Elderly individuals, especially those experiencing age-related cognitive decline or early signs of conditions such as dementia.

People with neurodegenerative diseases: Those with Alzheimer's, Parkinson's, or other neurological disorders that affect cognitive function.

Individuals recovering from brain injuries: Those who have suffered from strokes, traumatic brain injuries, or other incidents affecting brain health.

Anyone looking to maintain or enhance cognitive abilities can benefit from exercises that promote brain health and neuroplasticity, even without significant cognitive decline.

In summary, neurocognitive stimulation therapy is a powerful, non-invasive method for improving cognitive functions and promoting brain health. It offers a range of benefits, from slowing the progression of cognitive decline to enhancing the quality of life for individuals with mental challenges. The brain isn't a muscle, but like one, it thrives on regular exercise—challenging it with learning, creativity, and connection helps keep it strong, resilient, and vibrant.

# CHAPTER 5

# The Importance of Neurocognitive Therapy In Daily Practice

Neurocognitive therapy (NCT) is a specialized form of treatment designed to enhance cognitive functioning through targeted interventions. As the world's population ages and cognitive conditions such as Alzheimer's disease, Parkinson's disease, and other neurodegenerative disorders become increasingly prevalent, neurocognitive therapy plays a vital role in improving both the quality of life and the functional capabilities of individuals with cognitive decline.

Neurocognitive therapy addresses issues such as memory, attention, executive function, and problem-solving skills, which are essential for day-to-day living. The importance of neurocognitive therapy lies in its ability to help patients maintain cognitive function for as long as possible, reduce the impact of cognitive decline, and improve emotional well-being.

## Enhancing Cognitive Functioning

One of the primary goals of neurocognitive therapy is to help individuals maintain or improve their cognitive abilities. Cognitive functions such as memory, attention, and executive function are integral to daily life. Neurocognitive therapy utilizes various techniques, including mental training, stimulation exercises, and brain games, to target specific cognitive skills that may be deteriorating.

Memory training exercises are commonly employed in neurocognitive therapy to improve both short-term and long-term memory. Through repetitive tasks such as memorization drills, word associations, and recall exercises, individuals can strengthen their memory retention abilities. These tasks encourage neuroplasticity, which refers to the brain's ability to reorganize itself by forming new neural connections. Cognitive exercises that stimulate different areas of the brain can help individuals regain the ability to retain new information or recall past events more effectively.

Attention and concentration are also fundamental cognitive skills that NCT aims to improve. Attention training techniques may include exercises that focus on selective attention (the ability to focus on one stimulus while ignoring others) or sustained attention (the ability to maintain focus on a task over an extended period). Cognitive exercises, such as puzzles and concentration games, can challenge individuals to improve their focus and mental stamina. With a structured and personalized approach, neurocognitive therapy can help patients regain control over their cognitive abilities and restore confidence in their mental functioning.

## Delaying the Progression of Neurodegenerative Diseases

Neurodegenerative diseases like Alzheimer's disease, Parkinson's disease, and dementia are characterized by progressive cognitive decline. While these conditions often cannot be fully cured, neurocognitive therapy plays a crucial role in slowing their progression and alleviating symptoms. Regular engagement in neurocognitive training exercises has been shown to delay the onset of severe cognitive impairment and enhance overall well-being.

For patients with Alzheimer's disease, for example, research has indicated that cognitive stimulation programs can slow the decline in memory, reasoning, and language abilities. By consistently challenging the brain with cognitive tasks and exercises, individuals with Alzheimer's disease can strengthen neural networks, maintain mental agility, and reduce feelings of frustration and confusion. Such therapeutic interventions often provide significant benefits to patients and their families by enabling the individual to maintain their independence for longer. Parkinson's disease, which affects movement and cognition, also benefits from neurocognitive therapy. Cognitive difficulties in Parkinson's disease can include issues with attention, memory, and problem-solving, and neurocognitive therapy addresses these challenges by incorporating both motor and cognitive exercises into therapy. Combining physical exercises with mental stimulation promotes overall brain health and helps improve the patient's quality of life.

## Emotional and Psychological Benefits

In addition to its cognitive benefits, neurocognitive therapy offers significant emotional and psychological advantages. Cognitive decline can lead to feelings of helplessness, frustration, and depression, especially when individuals become aware of their cognitive limitations.

Neurocognitive therapy helps mitigate these feelings by promoting mental engagement and providing structured routines that enhance self-esteem and emotional well-being.

Patients engaged in neurocognitive therapy often report feeling empowered and in control of their cognitive abilities, even in the face of cognitive decline. This emotional boost is essential for maintaining a positive outlook and promoting mental resilience. Additionally, the therapeutic process itself can reduce anxiety and depression, which are common among individuals experiencing cognitive decline. Engaging in cognitive exercises in a supportive and encouraging environment helps combat feelings of isolation and promotes social engagement.

Research suggests that social interaction during neurocognitive therapy is also a key component in enhancing emotional well-being. Group therapy sessions, where individuals participate in cognitive exercises together, allow patients to form connections and share experiences, which can be both emotionally fulfilling and motivational. Such interactions not only strengthen cognitive skills but also foster a sense of community and support.

## Supporting Caregivers and Family Members

Neurocognitive therapy also plays a critical role in supporting caregivers and family members of individuals with cognitive impairments. Cognitive decline often affects not only the individual but also their loved ones, who may become overwhelmed with the challenges of caregiving. By slowing the progression of cognitive decline and helping individuals maintain their independence for longer, neurocognitive therapy can reduce the burden on caregivers.

Additionally, neurocognitive therapy provides caregivers with practical strategies to better support their loved ones. This includes techniques for encouraging cognitive engagement, helping patients stay organized, and managing behavioral symptoms such as agitation or confusion. Caregiver education programs that complement neurocognitive therapy allow family members to gain a deeper understanding of cognitive conditions and offer more effective care. For example, caregivers are often taught strategies to assist with memory recall, organize daily activities, and promote routines that help maintain cognitive function. These supportive measures can reduce stress, improve communication between caregivers and patients, and enhance the overall caregiving experience.

## The Role of Neuroplasticity in Recovery

Neuroplasticity is the brain's inherent ability to reorganize itself, create new neural connections, and compensate for injury or dysfunction. Neurocognitive therapy capitalizes on this ability by engaging individuals in exercises designed to stimulate and strengthen specific areas of the brain. Neuroplasticity is particularly important for those recovering from brain injuries, strokes, or other conditions that affect cognitive abilities.

For individuals who have experienced a traumatic brain injury, neurocognitive therapy can facilitate the reorganization of brain networks and help improve cognitive functions affected by the injury. By engaging in therapeutic activities that stimulate neuroplasticity, patients can regain skills such as attention, memory, and executive function, all of which are essential for everyday life.

Neuroplasticity is not limited to those recovering from brain injuries or neurodegenerative diseases; it is an essential process for everyone. Neurocognitive therapy encourages individuals to regularly challenge their brains, even in the absence of cognitive decline, to promote long-term brain health and reduce the risk of future cognitive impairment.

## Consistent Cognitive Care Made Easy

Incorporating neurocognitive exercises into daily life doesn't have to feel like a chore—it can be woven naturally into routines in ways that are both meaningful and enjoyable. Start by anchoring simple brain-boosting activities to tasks you already do, such as doing a crossword puzzle with your morning coffee, practicing a few minutes of mindful breathing before bed, or listening to an audiobook while walking. Rotate activities to stimulate different areas of the brain—try memory games one day, problem-solving challenges the next, and then something creative like drawing or storytelling. Keeping a small journal to track what you've done not only builds consistency but also offers a satisfying sense of progress.

The key to staying consistent is to make the exercises feel like play, not pressure. Turn brain workouts into social moments—invite a friend to a trivia night, teach someone a new recipe from memory, or join an online puzzle group. Add novelty by trying brain training apps, switching up routines, or learning a new language or musical instrument in short, manageable doses. When the activities spark curiosity or laughter, you're more likely to return to them daily. The goal isn't perfection but presence—keeping your brain curious, connected, and joyfully challenged each day.

## Conclusion

Neurocognitive therapy is a valuable tool for individuals experiencing cognitive decline or seeking to maintain their cognitive abilities. Through targeted interventions, cognitive exercises, and therapeutic approaches, neurocognitive therapy enhances cognitive functioning, helps slow the progression of neurodegenerative diseases, and empowers individuals to lead more independent and fulfilling lives, contributing to their overall well-being. Fostering neuroplasticity enables the brain to adapt and reorganize itself, offering hope to individuals recovering from brain injuries and cognitive impairments. The importance of neurocognitive therapy extends beyond the patient to caregivers and families, providing support and education to enhance their experience and strengthen their caregiving capabilities.

# CHAPTER 6

# SPARK© Neurocognitive Model of Care

First, let's define what SPARK© *is* at its core.

- The SPARK© Neurocognitive Model of Care is a program designed to enhance quality of life by improving social and emotional well-being, providing caregiver education and guidance, creating *person-centered care planning*, and stimulating sensory receptors through neurocognitive exercises.

**The pillars of SPARK:**

S = Sensory Stimulation
P = Personalized Routines
A = Active Engagement
R = Reflective Support
K = Kindness-based Caregiving

The SPARK© Neurocognitive Model of Care was developed by Benchmark Nursing Solutions founder Lisa A. Greenlee for families and caregivers of those affected by Alzheimer's and Dementia. It makes person-centered care planning with cognitive exercise central.

SPARK© combines education, caregiver support, care planning, and neurocognitive exercises to help improve patient outcomes and support living well throughout their disease process.
Damage caused by a stroke is unique to each individual, as is the recovery process. There is no one-size-fits-all plan. After a stroke, the neural pathways for storing, retrieving, and processing information can become altered, and during recovery, new neural pathways are formed. The brain often requires assistance and stimulation as it adapts to these cognitive changes.

Neurocognitive exercises and cueing help the brain re-route, rewire, and adapt, creating new neural pathways. Neurocognitive therapy is an integral aspect of the patient's treatment plan to help improve attention span and concentration. Additionally, neurocognitive therapy helps enhance auditory & visual processing, as well as memory. Individuals can experience high levels of anxiety from simple, everyday tasks; however, as brain function improves, patients develop a greater sense of security, and their anxieties lessen.

As we previously learned, neural plasticity refers to the nervous system's ability to change its activity in response to stimuli. A fascinating aspect of motor neurons is their ability to modify and strengthen the effects of synaptic transmission. And while the brain is not a muscle, we must treat it like one and help our patients enhance it with neurocognitive stimulation.

The neurocognitive exercises demonstrated later in the book help improve critical thinking skills through visual and auditory stimulation. These exercises become part of the patient's daily practice to enhance executive function and reduce anxiety, as well as alleviate feelings of being lost in a fog. By helping to reduce stress, patients experience greater emotional stability, making it easier for them to navigate challenging times.

Traditional care plans often place a greater emphasis on physical health, focusing on medications, mobility, and safety, while emotional and cognitive needs are sometimes overlooked. The SPARK© Neurocognitive Model of Care shifts this approach by recognizing that neurocognitive therapy, enrichment activities, and meaningful socialization are equally essential to overall well-being. By treating the mind, body, and spirit as interconnected, this model supports not only functional health but also emotional resilience, dignity, and joy throughout the care journey.

**For the Post-Stroke Patient**

Neurocognitive exercises are also beneficial for post-stroke patients. Damage caused by a stroke is unique to each individual, as is the recovery process and there is no one-size-fits-all plan. After a stroke, the neural pathways for storing, retrieving, and processing information can become altered, and during recovery, new neural pathways are formed. The brain often requires assistance and stimulation as it adapts to these cognitive changes.

Neurocognitive exercises play a vital role in the rehabilitation journey for post-stroke patients, targeting the brain's ability to rewire itself—a concept known as neuroplasticity. These exercises can include memory games, attention drills, problem-solving tasks, and language-based challenges that stimulate different areas of the brain affected by the stroke. When tailored to the individual's specific deficits and strengths, these mental workouts can help restore lost functions, reinforce new neural connections, and support emotional resilience. Even small, consistent efforts—like recalling daily schedules, engaging in simple math, or using naming apps—can contribute to strengthening cognitive pathways and improving day-to-day functionality.

Routine practice is essential for meaningful progress, as repetition helps embed cognitive skills and create new habits that compensate for what was lost. Just as physical therapy strengthens muscles, regular brain exercises can gradually rebuild mental agility, improve mood, and increase independence. Patients who engage daily—even in short bursts—often report better focus, confidence, and communication. Integrating these practices into a daily routine, ideally in coordination with occupational or speech therapy, ensures that cognitive recovery becomes a consistent part of the healing process rather than a sporadic effort. Over time, this steady engagement can significantly enhance quality of life and may even lead to partial or full recovery of certain cognitive abilities.

# CHAPTER 7

# Strategies for Caregivers

Caring for a loved one with Alzheimer's or dementia presents unique challenges that require patience, adaptability, and compassion. This document outlines key strategies that caregivers can implement to provide effective and empathetic care while ensuring their well-being.

## Establishing a Routine

Creating a structured daily routine can help reduce confusion and anxiety for individuals with dementia. Consistent schedules for meals, medication, and activities provide a sense of security and stability. Simple cues, such as using visual aids or reminders, can further reinforce the routine and promote a sense of stability and predictability.

## Effective Communication Techniques

Communicating with someone with dementia requires clear, simple, and reassuring language. Caregivers should:

- Use short sentences and simple words.
- Maintain eye contact and a calm tone.
- Avoid arguing or correcting unnecessarily.
- Offer choices instead of open-ended questions to reduce confusion.

## Creating a Safe and Supportive Environment

A dementia-friendly environment minimizes hazards and enhances the person's ability to navigate their space independently. Considerations include:

- Removing tripping hazards such as loose rugs and clutter.
- Installing grab bars and adequate lighting.
- Using locks or alarms on doors and windows is recommended if wandering is a concern.
- Labeling drawers, rooms, or frequently used items to assist with recognition.

## Managing Behavioral Changes

Individuals with Alzheimer's or dementia may exhibit agitation, aggression, or repetitive behaviors. Strategies to manage these include:

- Identifying triggers and addressing underlying causes, such as hunger, pain, or overstimulation, is crucial.
- Redirecting attention with calming activities such as music, art, or gentle exercise.
- Practicing reassurance through a calm presence and soothing words.
- Touch therapy, such as a gentle hand massage or reassuring touch on the shoulder, can help calm agitation in Alzheimer's patients by providing comfort, reducing anxiety, and fostering a sense of connection.

## Encouraging Meaningful Activities

Engaging individuals in activities they enjoy can help maintain cognitive function and emotional well-being.
Activities should be tailored to their abilities and interests, such as:

- Simple arts and crafts projects.
- Listening to familiar music.
- Gentle physical exercises like stretching or walking.
- Gardening or tending to small plants.
- Reminiscence Therapy & Conversation Cue.

## Nutrition and Hydration

Maintaining proper nutrition and hydration is crucial for individuals with dementia, as they may forget to eat or drink. Caregivers can:

- Provide small, nutrient-rich meals throughout the day.
- Offer easy-to-eat, finger-friendly foods.
- Ensure adequate water intake with reminders and flavored options, such as herbal teas.
- Set the stage with gentle music and allow dining to be a calming and pleasurable experience.

## Managing Caregiver Stress and Seeking Support

Caring for someone with Alzheimer's or dementia can be emotionally and physically demanding. To prevent burnout, caregivers should:

- Take breaks and seek respite care when needed.
- Join support groups for shared experiences and emotional support.
- Practice self-care through activities such as exercise, meditation, or hobbies.
- Ask for help from family, friends, or professional caregivers when necessary.

## Understanding the Progression of the Disease

Alzheimer's and dementia progress through distinct stages, and understanding these changes enables caregivers to adapt effectively. Individuals in the early stages may require reminders and minimal assistance, whereas those in later stages may necessitate full-time care and support.
Being informed about these stages allows caregivers to plan and adjust their approach accordingly.

## Utilizing Professional Resources

Caregivers do not have to navigate this journey alone. Seeking help from healthcare professionals, memory care specialists, and community organizations can provide essential guidance and support. Local Alzheimer's associations and online resources offer valuable tools for managing care effectively.

## Legal and Financial Planning

Early planning for legal and financial matters is essential. Caregivers should:

- Discuss power of attorney and healthcare directives with their loved ones while they can still participate in decision-making.
- Explore long-term care options and financial assistance programs.
- Keep important documents organized and accessible.

# CHAPTER 8

# Helpful Tools

Caring for someone with Alzheimer's or dementia requires patience, flexibility, and the right tools to support both the caregiver and the person living with the disease. As cognitive changes progress, daily tasks can become more complex, and behavioral symptoms may arise.
Fortunately, many practical tools and strategies can help caregivers create a safer, calmer, and more structured environment while also reducing their stress.

Memory aids and visual cues are invaluable in early to moderate stages. Labeling cabinets, using calendars, dry-erase boards, or digital reminder systems can help preserve independence and minimize confusion. Familiar photo albums, memory books, and storyboards are also great tools for prompting conversation and emotional connection through reminiscence. For some, voice-activated assistants can provide simple reminders for medications or appointments in a soothing and repeatable way.

Safety-focused technology also plays a vital role. Door alarms, bed alarms, motion sensors, stove shut-off devices, and GPS tracking watches offer peace of mind and can prevent accidents or wandering. Adaptive tools, such as weighted utensils, spill-proof cups, and dressing aids, also support day-to-day comfort and dignity as fine motor skills or coordination decline.

Ultimately, caregivers themselves require support tools to maintain their strength and well-being. Respite services, caregiver support groups, mobile apps for medication tracking or symptom journaling, and educational resources all empower caregivers to stay organized, supported, and informed. No one should walk this journey alone—and with the right tools in hand, both the caregiver and the person they love can experience more moments of peace, connection, and quality of life.

## Large-Print Calendar or Memory Calendar
Visual aid for appointments, birthdays, and family visits. Use color codes or stickers for clarity.

## Shower/Bathing Schedule
A weekly chart with set days for personal care. Reduces confusion and builds routine.

## Memory Clocks
Digital clocks that show full date, day, and time (e.g., "Tuesday Morning, April 15").

## Memory Boards
Memory boards can be a powerful tool for individuals living with Alzheimer's and other forms of dementia. By displaying familiar photos, names, and simple cues, these boards help spark recognition, support communication, and reinforce a sense of identity and connection with loved ones.

## Activity Cards or Brain Games Kit
Light puzzles, songs, or calming activities support mental stimulation. Store neurocognitive exercise activities in a designated container or box for easy access.

## Color-Coded Labels for Home Items
Labels or icons to help locate essentials, such as clothing, dishes, or medication.

## Visual Meal Plan or Food Tracker
Use photos or icons to guide healthy meals throughout the week.

## Exercise or Walking Schedule
A gentle routine with light physical activity—walking, stretching, or gardening.

## Wandering – Safe Return Devices
Wandering is a common and potentially dangerous behavior in individuals with Alzheimer's and other forms of dementia. Safe return devices—such as GPS-enabled wearables, ID bracelets, and location-tracking services—can provide peace of mind by helping caregivers quickly locate a loved one who has wandered. These tools not only enhance safety but also support greater independence, allowing individuals to engage with their environment while minimizing risk.

## Anti-Choking Device
You can purchase an antichoking device online. It should be kept in a designated location in the home for emergency use. All family and staff members should be aware of its location.

## Falls Prevention Equipment
Fall prevention is a critical aspect of dementia care, as individuals with Alzheimer's are at increased risk due to changes in balance, coordination, and judgment. Equipment such as grab bars, non-slip mats, bed and chair alarms, and motion-sensor lighting can significantly reduce the risk of falls at home. Mobility aids, such as walkers with stabilizers and fall detection devices, also enhance safety while supporting continued movement and independence.

## Home Safety Modifications:

- Grab bars – Installed in bathrooms and near beds or chairs to assist with stability.

- Non-slip mats or strips – Used in showers, bathtubs, and on smooth flooring to prevent slipping.

- Handrails – Placed along hallways and staircases for added support.

- Raised toilet seats with armrests – To facilitate safe transitions on and off the toilet

## Mobility Aids:

- Walkers with wheels and brakes – Offer stable mobility, especially for those with gait issues.

- Rollators (4-wheel walkers) – Include a seat and storage for rest and convenience.

- Canes with quad bases – Provide greater balance than single-point canes.

## Monitoring & Alert Systems:

- Bed and chair alarms – Alert caregivers when a person attempts to get up unassisted.

- Fall detection devices – Worn on the wrist or neck, these alert caregivers or emergency services automatically after a fall.

- Motion-sensor night lights – Illuminate walkways when movement is detected, reducing the risk of nighttime falls.

## Flooring and Furniture:

- Low-pile carpeting or secure rugs – Reduce trip hazards and cushion falls.

- Hip protectors – Padded garments that help prevent fractures in the event of a fall.

## Audio/Visual Remote Monitoring

Audio-visual monitoring devices can offer an added layer of safety and reassurance for individuals living with Alzheimer's. These tools allow caregivers to observe movement, detect falls, and monitor behavior patterns without being intrusive, helping to maintain the individual's dignity and independence. Many systems also offer real-time alerts and two-way communication, enabling quick response during emergencies and supporting around-the-clock care, even from a distance.

## Telephone Safety

Ex. TeleCalm is a specialized phone service designed to support individuals living with Alzheimer's and dementia by providing a safer, more straightforward way to stay connected. It helps prevent common risks such as scam calls, repeated dialing, and late-night calling while allowing trusted family and friends to reach their loved ones without disruption. With features tailored to the unique needs of dementia care, TeleCalm promotes independence, reduces caregiver stress, and enhances communication without compromising safety.

## Emergency Packet

For emergency medical technicians and hospital ER staff. Emergency packets are often kept on the face of the fridge. Emergency responders usually know where to look for these items. On the following three pages, you'll find a usable Emergency Packet. Complete each question and place the packet in an envelope, affixed to the front or side of your refrigerator, clearly marked
*"Emergency Packet for First Responders"*.

# CHAPTER 9

# Emergency Packets

Patient Name: _____

Date of Birth: _____

Address: _____

Phone Number: _____

Primary Language: _____

Preferred Name/Nickname: _____

## *In Case of Emergency, Call:*

1. Primary Support Person
Name: _____

Relationship: _____

Phone (Mobile): _____ Phone (Work/Home): _____

2. Secondary Support Person
Name: _____

Relationship: _____

Phone (Mobile): _____ Phone (Work/Home): _____

3. Primary Care Physician or Specialist
Name: _____

Practice Name: _____ Phone: _____

After-Hours Number: _____

4. Neurologist / Memory Care Specialist (if
different) Name: _____ Phone: _____

## *Preferred Hospital & Medical Info:*

Preferred Hospital: _____

Insurance Provider: _____

Policy Number: _____

## *Legal / Safety Information:*

Healthcare Power of Attorney (POA):

Name: _____

Phone: _____

## *Advance Directives / DNR Status:*
- ☐ On file in home
- ☐ On file with physician
- ☐ Copy attached

Wanders or Elopes? ☐ Yes ☐ No

Important Safety Info:

_____

_____

## *Additional Notes for First Responders:*

- The patient may be disoriented, anxious, or nonverbal during stress.

- Please speak calmly and avoid correcting memory errors.

- Familiar objects (photo, music, caregiver voice) may help calm.

- Has difficulty with: _____

- Comforted by: _____

| Active Diagnosis | Past Surgeries |
|---|---|
|  |  |
|  |  |
|  |  |
|  |  |

**Allergies:**_____

_____

## Medication Profile

| Medication Name | Dosage | Route | Admin. Time |
|---|---|---|---|
| Ex. Lisinopril HCTZ | 20/25 mg | 1 tab by mouth | Daily in am |
| | | | |
| | | | |
| | | | |
| | | | |
| | | | |
| | | | |
| | | | |
| | | | |
| | | | |
| | | | |
| | | | |
| | | | |
| | | | |
| | | | |
| | | | |
| | | | |

# CHAPTER 10

# Mini Cog Test for Tracking Changes

The Mini-Cog is not a diagnostic tool and is used by a nurse care manager, dementia care specialist, or another skilled clinician to gauge a baseline level of cognition and track changes over time.

Tracking changes in a person's cognition is a crucial aspect of delivering responsive, person-centered dementia care. Alzheimer's and other forms of dementia are progressive, and the needs of an individual can shift gradually or suddenly over time. By consistently observing and documenting changes—such as increased confusion, difficulty following instructions, new safety concerns, or changes in mood or behavior—caregivers can adjust interventions and daily routines to better support the individual's evolving abilities.

Cognitive tracking not only helps caregivers respond to challenges as they arise, but it also provides important insight into patterns and triggers. For example, noting that a person becomes more agitated in the late afternoon may point to sundowning, allowing caregivers to implement calming strategies or adjust the day's structure. Suppose memory lapses become more frequent or new behaviors emerge. In that case, these may signal that the person has progressed to a different stage of the disease, prompting a reassessment of their care plan, environment, and support systems.

Additionally, clear records of cognitive changes enable healthcare providers and family members to make informed decisions. Whether it's adjusting medications, considering assistive devices, or evaluating the need for additional in-home support or a higher level of care, this information ensures decisions are proactive rather than reactive. Tracking cognition isn't just clinical—it's a compassionate act. It helps preserve dignity, anticipate needs, and deliver care that honors the individual's journey with understanding and intention.

Below is an example of the SPARK© Mini Cog tool.

# SPARK©
## Mini-Cog

The SPARK© Mini Cog is not a diagnostic tool and is only used by a nurse, a care manager, a certified dementia care specialist, or other skilled clinician to gauge a baseline level of cognition and track changes over time.

1. Remember these 3 words. You will be asked to repeat them in a few minutes.
   a. Captain | Garden | Picture

2. Put the numbers on the clock where they belong. Then set the hands to fifteen minutes past ten. 2 pts.

3. What were the three words you were asked to remember?                    ( 3 pts )

   i.   1._____
   ii.  2._____
   iii. 3._____

4.  Put an X over the shape that is larger?                              ( 1 pt )

5.  Connect the shapes that are alike.                                   ( 1 pt )

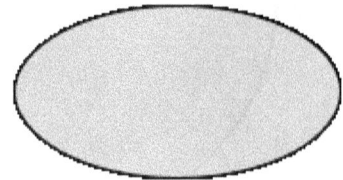

6.  Name as many animals as you can in thirty seconds. I will let you know when to
    start.

                                                                         ( 3 pts )

        ☐  1-5
        ☐  6-10
        ☐  10-15

Client Name:        _____
Date:               _____
Total points:       _____

# CHAPTER 11

# Care Plans for Alzheimer's & Dementia Patients

## Person-Centered Care Plans

A well-designed care plan is crucial for providing consistent, safe, and effective support to individuals who require assistance with daily living activities. It gives explicit instructions tailored to the specific needs, preferences, and routines of the person receiving care, enabling unlicensed or unskilled caregivers to deliver reliable and compassionate support. By outlining tasks such as personal hygiene, mobility assistance, meal preparation, and medication reminders, a care plan minimizes confusion, reduces the risk of errors, and promotes the individual's comfort and dignity.

Following a daily care plan is essential for caregivers, as it serves as both a practical guide and an emotional anchor amidst the demands of caregiving. With numerous moving parts in a typical day—medication schedules, hygiene routines, nutritional needs, mobility support, cognitive stimulation, and emotional reassurance—it becomes easy to overlook or unintentionally minimize critical aspects of care. A structured care plan helps prevent this by providing a clear, organized roadmap that outlines each task and its timing, thereby reducing the mental load of decision-making in the moment. It also allows caregivers to anticipate needs rather than react to them, which is vital in promoting consistency, safety, and dignity for the person receiving care.

By following a daily plan, caregivers are less likely to miss essential interventions, such as adjusting schedules to prevent pressure sores or providing hydration to reduce the risk of confusion or urinary tract infections.

Beyond meeting physical needs, care plans also incorporate moments of connection, rest, and routine that help preserve quality of life. Importantly, care plans provide documentation and accountability, making it easier for team members or family to step in, communicate effectively, and work collaboratively. In short, a daily care plan is not just a checklist—it is a lifeline that ensures the caregiver stays grounded, intentional, and attuned to the evolving needs of the person in their care.

## Care Plans for those with Alzheimer's & Dementia:

☐ Cognitive Support Plan

☐ Social Emotional Support Plan (for increased enrichment & socialization)

☐ Behavioral Management Plan (agitation, aggression, & anxiety)

☐ Personal Care and Hygiene Plan

☐ Nutrition and Hydration Plan

☐ Safety and Fall Prevention Plan

☐ Medication Management Plan

## Cognitive Support Plan

Implementing cognitive therapy exercises, reminiscence therapy, music therapy, and reality orientation techniques.

- Incorporate games, puzzles, word, and math problems into daily activities.

- Introduce sensory stimulation tools.

- Incorporate music therapy into daily activities, especially when dining.

- Take a walk down memory lane together.

- Provide orientation when necessary. Orient to time of day, day of the week, month, and year.

- It's not about getting the right answer or finishing the puzzle—it's about engaging your mind in the process, because the real benefit comes from using your brain along the way.

- Positive reinforcement, like offering praise or encouragement, helps build confidence and motivation, making the person feel valued and more willing to participate.

## Social and Emotional Support Plan

Encouraging social interaction, providing companionship, and supporting emotional well-being.

- Encourage Meaningful Social Interaction – Engage in conversations, family visits, or group activities to help reduce feelings of isolation.

- Use Gentle Reassurance – Offer comfort with a calm voice, physical touch, and positive affirmations.

- Validate Their Feelings – Acknowledge emotions rather than correcting or dismissing them.

- Engage in Familiar Activities – Encourage hobbies like music, art, or gardening to foster joy and connection.

- Create a Calm and Safe Environment – Reduce noise and distractions to ease anxiety and confusion.

- Maintain a Routine – Consistency in daily activities provides security and reduces stress.

- Provide Simple Choices – Offering limited, easy options empowers independence and confidence.

- Use Visual and Verbal Cues – Support communication with pictures, gestures, and clear, short sentences.

- Encourage Physical Touch – Holding hands, hugs, or a gentle pat on the shoulder can provide comfort.

- Support Caregiver Well-being – Encourage caregivers to seek support groups, respite care, and engage in self-care to provide the best emotional support for their loved ones.

## Behavioral Management Plan

Addressing agitation, aggression, and anxiety through non-pharmacological interventions.

### *Behavioral Management Strategies For Agitation & Aggression*

- Identify Triggers – Observe patterns to determine what causes agitation (e.g., pain, hunger, loud noises, unfamiliar environments).

- Stay Calm and Reassuring – Use a gentle tone and relaxed body language to avoid escalating the situation.

- Redirect Attention – Shift focus to a favorite activity, object, or conversation.

- Maintain a Consistent Routine – Predictability reduces confusion and frustration.

- Avoid Arguing or Confrontation – Instead, validate feelings and provide comfort.

- Ensure Basic Needs Are Met – Hunger, thirst, discomfort, or fatigue can contribute to aggression.

- Modify the Environment – Reduce overstimulation by controlling noise levels, lighting, and clutter.

- Use Nonverbal Communication – Gentle touch, eye contact, and smiling can help soothe agitation.
- Provide Meaningful Activities – Engaging in hobbies or simple tasks can reduce frustration.

- Use Medications as a Last Resort – Only if prescribed by a doctor.

## *Behavioral Management Strategies For Anxiety*

- Create a Calm Environment – Soft lighting, familiar objects, and quiet spaces can be soothing.

- Encourage Physical Activity – Walking, stretching, or simple exercises help reduce restlessness.

- Use Reassuring Language – Offer comfort by saying, "You're safe" or "I'm here to help."

- Engage in Relaxing Activities – Music therapy, aromatherapy, or deep breathing exercises can help.

- Limit Stimulants – Reduce your intake of caffeine and sugar, especially in the evening.

- Provide a Security Object – A familiar blanket, stuffed animal, or photo can bring comfort.

- Simplify Communication – Use short, clear sentences and avoid overwhelming instructions.

- Offer Distractions – Encourage participation in activities such as puzzles, reading, or sorting objects to help ease anxious thoughts.

- Validate Emotions – Acknowledge feelings without dismissing them, saying, "I understand this is hard."

- Monitor for underlying medical issues, including pain or infection.

## Personal Care and Hygiene Plan

Assisting with bathing, dressing, and grooming while preserving dignity.

- Establish a Routine – Maintain a consistent daily schedule for bathing, dressing, and grooming to reduce confusion and anxiety.

- Use Simple Instructions – Give step-by-step verbal or visual cues to guide them through the process.

- Ensure a Safe Bathroom Setup – Install grab bars, non-slip mats, and a shower chair to prevent falls.

- Encourage Independence – Allow them to do as much as possible on their own, offering assistance only when needed.

- Choose Comfortable Clothing – Opt for easy-to-wear clothes with Velcro, elastic waistbands, or front closures.

- Maintain Oral Hygiene – Assist with brushing teeth or provide alternative options like mouthwash or floss picks.

- Be Patient and Reassuring – Use a calm tone and avoid rushing, as resistance can increase with frustration.

- Adapt Bathing Methods – If they resist showers, try sponge baths or allow them to assist with washing.

- Monitor for Skin Issues – Check for dryness, irritation, or infections, especially in areas prone to pressure sores.

- Make Hygiene Enjoyable – Play soothing music, use scented lotions, or allow them to choose their favorite soap to create a pleasant experience.

## Nutrition and Hydration Plan

Monitoring dietary intake, providing nutrient-rich meals, and preventing dehydration.

- Maintain a Routine – Serve meals at the same time each day to create consistency and encourage healthy eating habits.

- Offer Nutrient-Dense Foods – Provide meals that are high in protein, fiber, and vitamins.

- Make Eating Easy – Serve finger foods or pre-cut meals if using utensils becomes difficult.

- Encourage Hydration – Offer water, herbal teas, or flavored drinks regularly to prevent dehydration.

- Limit Processed and Sugary Foods – Reduce excess sugar and unhealthy fats to support brain health.

- Monitor for Chewing or Swallowing Issues – Provide soft, moist foods or thickened liquids if needed.

- Minimize Mealtime Distractions – Serve food in a quiet, well-lit environment to help focus on eating.

- Use Adaptive Utensils – Consider weighted utensils, non-slip plates, or cups with lids for easier eating and drinking.
- Make Mealtimes Enjoyable – Play soft music, engage in pleasant conversation, and avoid rushing.

- Watch for Weight Changes – Monitor appetite, weight loss, or gain, and adjust meals accordingly.

## Safety and Fall Prevention Plan

Ensuring a safe environment, using mobility aids, and reducing fall risks.

### *Tips to Prevent Falls*

- Ensure Proper Lighting – Use bright, even lighting in hallways, staircases, and bathrooms.

- Remove Clutter and Hazards – Keep walkways clear of cords, rugs, and furniture.

- Install Grab Bars and Handrails – Place them in bathrooms, stairways, and other necessary areas.

- Use Non-Slip Flooring – Add non-slip mats in wet areas and wear shoes with good traction.

- Encourage Safe Footwear – Avoid loose slippers or high heels; opt for sturdy, non-slip shoes.

- Promote Strength and Balance Exercises – Engage in activities like tai chi, yoga, or physical therapy.

- Monitor Medications – Be aware of potential side effects, such as dizziness, that may increase the risk of falls.

- Adjust Furniture and Seating – Ensure chairs and beds are at a safe height for easy sitting and standing.

- Encourage Proper Hydration and Nutrition – Dehydration and weakness can contribute to falls.

- Use Mobility Aids When Needed – Ensure canes, walkers, or wheelchairs are properly fitted.

## Medication Management Plan

As people age, they are more likely to develop chronic conditions that require regular and sometimes complex medication regimens. For seniors with memory concerns—whether from normal aging, mild cognitive impairment, or conditions like Alzheimer's disease or other forms of dementia—managing medications can become a significant and sometimes dangerous challenge.

One of the primary difficulties is remembering to take medications at the right times and in the correct doses. Many seniors are prescribed multiple medications, often with different schedules and instructions (e.g., take with food, avoid certain combinations, or take at bedtime). Memory impairment can lead to skipped doses, double doses, or taking the wrong medication entirely. These errors can have serious health consequences, including worsening of conditions, dangerous drug interactions, or even hospitalization.

Another challenge is organizing and tracking prescriptions. Seniors may struggle to understand medication labels, recognize pills by shape or color, or keep up with changes made by healthcare providers. Confusion can be compounded when medication regimens are altered—such as switching dosages or adding new drugs—without clear and repeated instructions.

This is why having a **safe, reliable, and easy-to-manage medication management system** is critically important.

Such a system reduces the risks of medication errors, ensures that medications are taken as prescribed, and helps catch potential problems early. It also provides peace of mind for caregivers and family members, knowing that their loved one is following their treatment plan consistently. A well-designed system—whether it involves a simple weekly pill organizer, digital reminders, or automated dispensing devices—can help maintain a senior's independence while also safeguarding their health.

Furthermore, a dependable system can enhance communication among seniors, caregivers, and healthcare providers. Accurate medication tracking enables better treatment decisions, reduces unnecessary emergency room visits, and contributes to a higher quality of life.

Ultimately, managing medications safely for seniors with memory concerns requires a combination of practical tools, professional oversight, and compassionate support. A thoughtfully chosen medication management system isn't just a convenience—it's a cornerstone of safe, effective, and dignified care.

Utilize your nurse care manager for administering prescribed medications, tracking side effects, and maintaining adherence.

## *The Rights of Medication Administration are:*

- Right Patient – If your team is caring for more than one person in a household, ensure the medication is given to the correct person by verifying the name on their medication bottles.

- Right Medication – Verify the medication name, strength, and expiration date to confirm they match the prescription.

- Right Dose – Administer the correct amount of medication as prescribed, measuring accurately to avoid overdosing or underdosing.

- Many healthcare personnel follow the Five or Seven Rights, which also include the principles of Right Time, Right Route, Right Documentation, and Right Reason.

Remember, a care plan is an essential guide for providing safe, consistent, and person-centered care, especially for individuals living with Alzheimer's or dementia. In the face of cognitive decline, where memory loss and confusion can compromise safety and well-being, a well-crafted care plan becomes the foundation of quality care. It ensures that the entire care team—whether professionals, family members, or support staff—has access to the same detailed, up-to-date information. This includes daily routines, medication management, behavior triggers, personal preferences, communication strategies, safety concerns, and emotional needs. When used consistently, a care plan prevents crucial tasks from being forgotten or overlooked, reducing caregiver stress and improving outcomes for the individual.

A structured care plan also acts as a powerful communication tool. By clearly documenting each component of care, all caregivers—regardless of shift or role—can align their efforts. This avoids gaps in care, duplicated tasks, or miscommunication that could lead to agitation, injury, or emotional distress for the person with dementia. It empowers the team to collaborate effectively, and it reassures families that their loved one's unique needs are being understood and honored. In settings where multiple caregivers are involved, the care plan provides continuity and consistency, which build trust and stability —two factors that are especially important in dementia care.

Routine is critical for individuals with Alzheimer's or other forms of dementia. Predictability brings comfort. When their world feels unfamiliar and disorienting, having a dependable rhythm to the day—knowing when meals will be served, when walks will happen, or how bedtime is prepared—helps reduce anxiety and behavioral symptoms. The care plan safeguards that structure. Even as symptoms progress, caregivers can use the plan to adapt routines thoughtfully, honoring the person's history and preferences while ensuring safety and dignity.

# DAILY CARE PLAN

**Day of the Week:** _____ **Today's Date:** _____

## PERSONAL CARE

- ☐ Morning bath/shower completed
- ☐ Deodorant applied
- ☐ Lotions, creams or protective powder applied
- ☐ Clean clothes donned
- ☐ Hair brushed or combed
- ☐ Oral hygiene completed

## MEALS PROVIDED

- ☐ Breakfast
- ☐ Lunch
- ☐ Dinner
- ☐ Snacks

## MEDICATION

- ☐ Yes, morning medicine was taken.
- ☐ Yes, afternoon medicine was taken.
- ☐ Yes, bedtime medicine was taken.

**Good fluid intake helps prevent dehydration.**

(coffee, tea, orange juice, apple juice, Ensure, water)

*place an X over each glass*

**Enrichment & Socialization** It is important that you engage in conversation throughout the day and evening to ensure emotional needs are being met and to help build trust for a healthy caregiver/client relationship.

## Exercise & Engagement

- ☐ I took a walk today | We exercised & practiced range of motion
- ☐ I read aloud from a book, magazine, or newspaper today
- ☐ We listened to music for relaxation and while dining
- ☐ We took a walk down memory lane through conversation

## Daily Reminders for Care Team

- ☐ Exercise contributes to good circulation.
- ☐ Keep the walker or wheelchair nearby for safety.
- ☐ Offer bathroom breaks every 2 hours and as needed.
- ☐ Ensure the patient or loved one is clean and dry at all times after toileting.
- ☐ Providing personal care helps individuals stay clean, dry, and free from breakdown.
- ☐ Assist with bedtime routine, providing verbal cues & assistance as needed.
- ☐ Toileting before bedtime helps empty the bladder, allowing for dry overnight sleep.
- ☐ Ensure they have clean undergarments before bed.
- ☐ If a bed alarm is in use, ensure it is in place and on to prevent nighttime falls.
- ☐ Report any concerns or changes in condition to family members.
- ☐ Know where emergency contacts and numbers are kept.
- ☐ Call 911 for medical emergencies.

## NOTES:

_____
_____
_____
_____
_____

## EMERGENCY CONTACT INFORMATION:

Name: _____     Name: _____

Relationship: _____     Relationship: _____

Telephone _____     Telephone _____

# Daily Care Plan Checklist

**Date** _____

## Morning (7:00 AM – 10:00 AM)

☐ Gently wake the person with a calm, familiar voice

☐ Assist with toileting and hygiene (brushing teeth, washing face)

☐ Administer morning medications

☐ Help with dressing (lay out simple clothing choices)

☐ Serve a healthy, familiar breakfast

☐ Encourage hydration (offer a glass of water)

☐ Engage in a light morning activity (e.g., a walk, music, or photo album)

## Mid-Morning (10:00 AM – 12:00 PM)

☐ Encourage a simple, engaging activity (e.g., folding towels, puzzles)

☐ Monitor for signs of confusion or agitation

☐ Offer a light snack and water

☐ Check for toileting needs

## Midday (12:00 PM – 2:00 PM)

☐ Prepare and serve lunch (small, manageable portions)

☐ Provide bathroom assistance

☐ Administer midday medications (if prescribed)

☐ Encourage rest or quiet time after lunch

## Afternoon (2:00 PM – 5:00 PM)

☐ Offer a simple, soothing activity (e.g., coloring, sorting objects)

☐ Play calming music or watch a familiar show

☐ Provide a snack and encourage fluids

☐ Reassure and redirect if they become confused or agitated

☐ Encourage a brief outdoor walk or sit in natural light if possible

## Evening (5:00 PM – 8:00 PM)

- ☐ Prepare and serve dinner (soft, easy-to-digest foods)
- ☐ Bathroom assistance
- ☐ Administer evening medications
- ☐ Begin winding down: turn off bright lights, lower volume and add a calming activity (e.g., reading aloud, soft music)

## Bedtime (8:00 PM – 10:00 PM)

- ☐ Assist with nighttime hygiene (toothbrushing, toileting)
- ☐ Help them into comfortable sleepwear
- ☐ Set up a calm sleep environment (dim lights, remove clutter
- ☐ Reassure and say goodnight with a consistent routine
- ☐ Ensure safety measures are in place (bed rails, night light, door alarm if needed)

## General Daily Reminders

- ☐ Maintain a calm, reassuring tone throughout the day
- ☐ Use short, clear instructions
- ☐ Maintain safety at all times
- ☐ Ensure client or loved one is clean and dry at all times
- ☐ Monitor for changes in condition

## Emergency Contact Information

Name: _____     Name: _____

Relationship: _____     Relationship: _____

Telephone _____     Telephone _____

# CHAPTER 12

# Strength, Stamina & Skilled Support

## The Physical Side of Dementia Care

While Alzheimer's and other forms of dementia are most commonly associated with memory and cognitive decline, the physical health and strength of a person living with dementia are just as essential to their safety, dignity, and overall quality of life. Maintaining mobility, balance, and stamina can significantly delay the need for higher levels of care, reduce the risk of falls, and improve emotional well-being. As dementia progresses, individuals often become more sedentary, fatigued, or hesitant in movement, which makes intentional support for physical function even more vital. Skilled services can be used for maintenance care to help individuals with Alzheimer's maintain mobility, communication abilities, and overall function, even when full recovery is not expected.

Good balance begins with strength and stamina. Weak leg muscles, an unsteady gait, and slower reaction times can lead to falls, one of the most common and dangerous risks in dementia care. Encouraging daily movement, even in small and supported ways, helps maintain the muscle tone, flexibility, and coordination necessary for stability. Activities such as walking short distances, performing seated exercises, engaging in stretching routines, or practicing simple range-of-motion tasks can help preserve physical function and increase individuals' confidence and capability in their bodies.

Caregivers should also be vigilant in observing and monitoring changes in gait, posture, and coordination. Shuffling feet, hesitation before stepping, favoring one side, or relying heavily on furniture for support can be early signs of decline in balance or strength. These changes may not be verbalized by the person experiencing them, but they speak volumes through their movement. A sudden increase in falls or near-falls, increased fatigue after basic tasks, or difficulty rising from a chair are red flags that should not be ignored.

When such signs appear—or ideally, before they do—it's important to involve skilled care providers who specialize in functional support. Physical therapists can help build strength and balance, design safe mobility routines, and recommend assistive devices when needed.

Occupational therapists assess how safely and independently a person can perform daily tasks and introduce strategies, equipment, or modifications to support activities such as dressing, bathing, eating, and toileting. Speech-language pathologists play a critical role as well, addressing not only communication challenges but also issues related to swallowing and cognition, both of which can decline as the disease progresses.

Bringing in these specialists early fosters a proactive approach to care. Therapy isn't just for recovery—it's also for preservation. It empowers individuals to hold onto their independence for as long as possible and gives caregivers confidence in knowing their loved one is supported from all angles—physically, emotionally, and cognitively. Regular check-ins with these providers can help track changes over time and ensure the care plan evolves in tandem with the individual's needs.

In the journey of dementia care, physical strength and balance often go unnoticed—until they're lost. But with mindful attention, gentle encouragement, and the involvement of skilled therapists, caregivers can help maintain function and prevent unnecessary decline. Supporting the body is just as sacred as supporting the mind, and when both are honored, we offer a fuller, more compassionate model of care.

## What to Do When You Notice Physical Decline and How to Involve Skilled Services

### 1. Pay Attention

- Keep an eye out for subtle or marked changes.

- Changes in gait (shuffling, limping, unsteady steps)

- Difficulty standing up from a chair or bed

- Increased fatigue after simple tasks

- Frequent falls or near-falls

- Trouble dressing, bathing, or feeding

- Slurred speech or coughing while eating

### 2. Communicate with the Primary Care Provider

- Share your concerns with the treating physician.

- Use specific examples ("Mom has fallen twice this week" or "Dad now takes much longer to stand from a chair").

- Request a referral for therapy services: Physical Therapy (PT), Occupational Therapy (OT), or Speech-Language Pathology (SLP).

### 3. Understand Which Service to Involve

- **Physical Therapy (PT):** For mobility, balance, fall prevention, strength, endurance, and assistive device assessment.

- **Occupational Therapy (OT):** For activities of daily living (ADLs), home safety, energy conservation, hand/arm coordination, and adaptive equipment.

- **Speech Therapy (SLP):** For communication support, swallowing difficulties, and cognitive therapy (such as memory, sequencing, and attention).

And remember, the primary care physician plays a key-role in guiding the direction of care by assessing the patient's condition and recommending skilled services, so don't be afraid to ask for help if you're unsure.

## 4. Request a Home Health Evaluation

- If the person qualifies (often due to recent decline or falls), ask the provider to order **home health services**.
- Home health agencies will send a nurse to the home to evaluate potential needs.

Most insurance plans, including Medicare, permit in-home skilled services when specific criteria are met. Skilled services include Nursing, physical therapy, occupational therapy, and Speech Therapy.

## 5. Be Proactive with Prevention

- Even if no urgent decline is noted, request preventive therapy assessments for safety checks, exercise guidance, or caregiver training to ensure ongoing support.

- Consider outpatient therapy if home health isn't appropriate but concerns remain.

## 6. Reassess the Care Plan

- Update the care plan with the therapist's recommendations.

- Incorporate exercises, home modifications, or equipment into daily routines.

- Educate all care partners and family members about new safety equipment and protocols.

## In Summary

Safety is always a priority in care, but it shouldn't come at the cost of activity and engagement. When individuals are encouraged to move—whether through gentle exercise, walking, or stretching—they often maintain their strength, balance, and independence for a more extended period. Regular physical activity also boosts mood, improves circulation, and supports brain health, making it a vital part of a well-rounded care plan that values both protection and vitality.

# CHAPTER 13

# Supporting a Spouse
# with Alzheimer's or Dementia

When your partner is diagnosed with Alzheimer's or dementia, life changes in profound ways. While every journey is unique, here is a gentle guide to help you navigate the emotional and practical challenges with compassion and strength.

## Emotional Support & Mindset

- **Grieve the Changes**
  It's natural to feel grief as you witness the slow shift in your loved one. This is called an *ambiguous loss*. Allow yourself to feel and express your emotions guilt-free.
- **Practice Patience**
  Their memory lapses or confusion are not a personal issue. Try not to correct or argue; instead, join them in their reality with empathy.
- **Celebrate Small Moments**
  Some days bring a smile, a familiar laugh, or a shared memory. These small moments are precious—hold onto them.

## Practical Care Tips

- **Establish Routines**
  Regular schedules reduce anxiety and help them feel more secure.
- **Offer Simple Choices**
  Avoid overwhelming them. Ask clear, limited-option questions like, "Would you like tea or coffee?"
- **Make the Home Safer**
  Install handrails, remove clutter, label rooms or drawers—simple adjustments make a big difference.

## Self-Care for the Caregiver

- **Ask for Help**
  You are not alone. Reach out to family, friends, or professionals for support. Even a short break can restore your energy.
- **Keep a Piece of Yourself**

Whether it's a hobby, journaling, your faith, or creative work, nurture your own identity and joy.

- **Learn in Small Steps**
  Stay informed about dementia, but don't overwhelm yourself. Knowledge brings confidence—take it one step at a time.

**You're Not Alone** – Joining a support group, whether online or in person, can make a significant difference. Others walking a similar path can offer insight, compassion, and sometimes, a bit of humor to light the way.

# CHAPTER 14

# For The Newly Diagnosed: You Are Not Alone

If you've just received a diagnosis of Alzheimer's or dementia, it's natural to feel fear, confusion, or even grief. But this is not the end of your story. Many people continue to live meaningful, connected lives in the early and middle stages of dementia.

## Give Yourself Time
You don't need to have all the answers right now. Allow yourself time to adjust and process the implications of this.

## Stay Connected
Let your loved ones support you. Isolation can increase fear; community and connection can ease it.

## Focus on What You Can Do
Your abilities and identity remain intact. Make decisions while you're able, explore new ways to stay engaged, and celebrate what you *can* do.

## The Power of Connection
After a new diagnosis of Alzheimer's or dementia, leaning on your social support network can provide comfort, strength, and practical help during a time of uncertainty. Friends, family, faith communities, and support groups can offer emotional reassurance, assist with daily tasks, and help you process the changes ahead. You don't have to face this journey alone—allow others to walk beside you.

## You Are Still You
A diagnosis does not diminish your worth, memories, or spirit. You are still loved, still valuable, still *you*.

## Put Your Own Plan in Place
After receiving an Alzheimer's or dementia diagnosis, it's important to put a clear care plan in place that reflects your values, preferences, and future wishes. This may include appointing a healthcare proxy, completing advance directives, and discussing long-term care goals with your loved ones and care team. Planning ahead ensures your voice is heard and respected, even if you are no longer able to communicate your decisions later on.

**With love and strength,** you are doing the most important work there is—loving someone through every season. Be gentle with them, and be just as gentle with yourself.

# CHAPTER 15

# Living in the Fog:
# Depression in Alzheimer's and Dementia

## From the Perspective of the Person Living with Dementia

It begins quietly. A forgotten name here, a missed appointment there. At first, it may seem like ordinary forgetfulness—something to laugh off. But as Alzheimer's or dementia progresses, the reality becomes harder to ignore. There's a creeping awareness that something fundamental is slipping away. It's not just memory—it's the sense of self, the ease of navigating the world, the once effortless ability to participate in conversation or complete simple tasks. This loss, both invisible and relentless, often leads to a deep emotional toll: depression.

For many individuals living with cognitive decline, depression can feel like a second diagnosis—a shadow that follows the memory loss. It may manifest as a loss of interest in previously enjoyed activities, withdrawal from family and friends, increased irritability, or even apathy. There can be moments of awareness and insight when the person knows something is wrong, and that awareness may be accompanied by waves of grief, fear, or helplessness.

Unlike classic depression, the emotional suffering in dementia is often masked or minimized. A person may not have the language to express what they're feeling, or they may become frustrated when their emotional state is misunderstood. Apathy—a lack of motivation and interest—is particularly common in dementia-related depression, and it is often misinterpreted as laziness or disengagement when it's actually a symptom of a neurochemical and emotional imbalance.

Depression can arise from many sources: fear of becoming a burden, disorientation in once-familiar spaces, social isolation, physical changes, or even medications. Sometimes, it's grief over the loss of independence or the subtle but significant changes in relationships. These emotional wounds can feel invisible, yet they cut deeply.

While people with dementia may not always be able to verbalize their inner struggles, they often feel them intensely. Offering consistent reassurance, emotional validation, and a gentle presence can provide a lifeline. Their world may be changing, but with understanding, structure, and support, they don't have to navigate it in despair.

# From the Caregiver's Perspective

Caregiving is a sacred and often solitary path, especially for those walking alongside someone with Alzheimer's or dementia. One of the most heart-wrenching challenges caregivers face is witnessing their loved one experience depression—an emotional heaviness that can cloud even their best days. As memory fades and cognitive functions decline, caregivers may find themselves mourning the person their loved one once was while trying to comfort the one they are now.

Depression in dementia is not always easy to recognize. Caregivers may notice changes in appetite, sleep, or personality—yet these shifts can easily be attributed to the progression of the disease itself. It takes careful attention to distinguish what may be a symptom of depression versus what's part of cognitive decline. A caregiver might hear their loved one say, "What's the point?" or notice they no longer want to go on walks or join family meals. These can be signs that depression is settling in.

But caregivers, too, are vulnerable to depression, often called "caregiver burnout" or "compassion fatigue." The emotional labor of providing daily care, managing appointments, responding to mood swings, and making difficult decisions can erode even the most resilient spirit. Many caregivers put their own needs aside, feeling guilty for expressing sadness or frustration. But those unspoken feelings accumulate, and without adequate support, caregivers can find themselves depleted and struggling to cope.

Addressing depression—for both the person with dementia and the caregiver—requires a multi-layered approach. Medical evaluation is critical, as there may be treatments (including antidepressants or mood stabilizers) that can help. Counseling or therapy can provide an outlet for both parties. Participating in structured daily routines, engaging in light physical activity, and preserving social interaction (even if limited) can also help lift the emotional fog.

Caregivers should not have to bear the weight of caregiving alone. Seeking out respite care, support groups, or family counseling can provide moments of rest and emotional anchoring. No one is meant to do this alone.

# Understanding the Overlap

Depression and dementia share many overlapping symptoms: apathy, low energy, poor concentration, and changes in appetite or sleep. This overlap can make it difficult to separate the two, but it is important to try. Left untreated, depression can accelerate cognitive decline, reduce quality of life, and undermine the gains of even the most well-designed care plans.

In early-stage dementia, depression may be more overt—sadness, crying spells, expressions of hopelessness. As the disease progresses, depression may become more behavioral: withdrawal, resistance to care, irritability, or agitation. Observing and documenting these shifts can help healthcare providers make better-informed decisions.

# Steps for Caregivers to Take

1. **Track changes**: Keep a journal to note your mood, behavior, appetite, and sleep. These notes can help professionals identify depressive patterns.

2. **Seek a professional evaluation**: Geriatric psychiatrists, neurologists, and primary care physicians can help assess whether depression is present and recommend treatment.

3. **Encourage engagement**: Even passive participation in music, art, or spiritual rituals can be uplifting. Focus on joy over productivity.

4. **Provide consistent reassurance**: The person may feel lost or frightened. Your calm, loving presence can be grounding.

## A Closing Reflection

Depression in Alzheimer's and dementia is not a character flaw or weakness—it is a valid, treatable part of the neurocognitive journey. For the person living with dementia, being seen, heard, and comforted can create emotional safety. For the caregiver, finding connection, rest, and support is not a luxury—it is essential for endurance.

Both roles—patient and caregiver—are marked by bravery. In a world that often overlooks the emotional toll of cognitive decline, choosing compassion, reaching for help, and holding onto moments of joy are acts of quiet courage.

# CHAPTER 16

# Honoring the Journey: When to Consider Memory Care

A family may consider transitioning a loved one to a memory care community, facility, or specialized unit within a multilevel care community when certain signs indicate that their cognitive decline requires more structured, specialized support than can be provided at home or in a general senior living setting. Here are some common reasons:

## When to Consider Memory Care:

1. **Increasing Safety Concerns**
   Frequent wandering, getting lost even in familiar places, forgetting to turn off appliances, or difficulty managing medications can create unsafe living situations.

2. **Progressive Cognitive Decline**
   When dementia or Alzheimer's disease progresses to the point where memory loss, confusion, or disorientation significantly interferes with daily functioning and quality of life.

3. **Behavioral Changes**
   Heightened anxiety, aggression, agitation, or paranoia that becomes difficult to manage without trained support.

4. **Decline in Personal Care**
   Inability to bathe, dress, or manage toileting independently, leading to hygiene issues or health complications, and nobody to assist with care.

5. **Caregiver Burnout**
   When caregiving demands exceed the emotional, physical, or financial capacity of family members and respite care is no longer enough.

6. **Structured Environment Needed**
   Individuals benefit from a daily routine, cognitive stimulation, and social engagement that memory care units are specifically designed to provide.

7.  **Medical Oversight Required**
    Coexisting medical conditions or complex medication regimens need monitoring by staff trained in dementia care.

8.  **Limited Support and Rising Costs of In-Home Care.** When the cost of providing adequate in-home care becomes unsustainable—or when reliable help is hard to find or coordinate—families may need to consider memory care. Memory care communities offer consistent, around-the-clock support that can often be more practical and cost-effective than trying to piece together services at home, especially as needs increase.

# CHAPTER 17

# Embracing Comfort: Knowing When to Welcome Hospice Support

## What is Hospice?

Hospice is a philosophy of care designed to support individuals who are facing a terminal illness, typically in the last six months of life, when curative treatments are no longer effective or desired. The focus shifts from curing the disease to enhancing quality of life, comfort, and dignity. Hospice care addresses the physical, emotional, and spiritual needs of both the person and their family. It is not about giving up; rather, it is about choosing how one wishes to live during the final stage of life, with an emphasis on compassionate presence, symptom management, and support for decision-making.

For individuals living with Alzheimer's disease or other forms of dementia, hospice can offer a layer of care that is both gentle and skilled. As dementia progresses into its later stages, individuals may lose the ability to communicate discomfort, eat independently, or respond to their environment. Hospice teams—often including nurses, aides, social workers, chaplains, and volunteers—work together to assess subtle signs of distress and provide personalized interventions. Families are not alone during this time. Hospice provides education, respite, and emotional support to caregivers, helping them feel more confident and less overwhelmed as they walk alongside their loved one. Far from being the end, hospice can become a space of peace, reconciliation, and deeply meaningful connection.

## How will Hospice help us in our journey?

Hospice care for individuals with Alzheimer's or other forms of dementia focuses on comfort, dignity, and quality of life during the advanced stages of the disease. It is typically considered when a physician determines that the individual has a life expectancy of six months or less if the disease follows its expected course. This type of care does not aim to cure the condition but instead provides pain management, emotional support, and assistance with daily activities, often in the home, a hospice facility, or a memory care community.

For dementia patients, hospice can be especially beneficial as it includes:

- Skilled care to manage agitation, infections, swallowing difficulties, and other complications common in late-stage dementia

- A multidisciplinary team—including nurses, social workers, chaplains, and aides—that supports both the patient and the family

- Respite care to give exhausted caregivers a break

- Bereavement services to help families cope with loss before and after death

Choosing hospice is not about giving up—it's about choosing peace, comfort, and meaningful support at the end of a long journey.

## When to call on Hospice

Deciding when to call on hospice can be one of the most challenging decisions families face during the progression of Alzheimer's or dementia. Hospice care is appropriate when the disease has reached an advanced stage, and curative treatments are no longer effective or desired. Signs that it may be time to consider hospice include significant weight loss, frequent infections, difficulty swallowing, increased confusion or agitation, and a general decline in physical functioning, such as inability to walk or sit without assistance. When these symptoms signal that the person's health is rapidly declining and their life expectancy is estimated to be six months or less, hospice can provide compassionate support focused on comfort and quality of life.

Hospice is not just about managing physical symptoms—it also offers emotional, spiritual, and practical support for both the individual and their family. If caregivers are feeling overwhelmed or burned out by the demands of daily care, hospice teams can step in to provide relief and guidance. They help manage complex symptoms like pain, anxiety, or agitation, often providing medications and therapies tailored specifically to the unique needs of dementia patients.

Additionally, hospice staff can assist families in navigating difficult decisions, offering counseling and resources to help prepare for the end-of-life journey.

Early involvement of hospice can improve quality of life by allowing the patient to remain in a familiar environment—whether at home or in a memory care setting—surrounded by loved ones and cared for by professionals trained in dementia care. Families are encouraged to reach out to hospice providers when they notice increased hospitalizations, frequent infections like pneumonia or urinary tract infections, or when basic care needs become too difficult to manage safely. In this way, hospice becomes a partner in care, ensuring dignity, comfort, and peace during the final chapter of life.

# CHAPTER 18

# Guidance for Mediating Family Dynamics Related to Care Decisions

Having an elder law attorney on your care team is not just about legal counsel—they become a trusted guide, offering compassionate support, clear direction in times of crisis, and ensuring every legal need is met with foresight and care.

Navigating care decisions for an aging loved one often brings families face-to-face with complex emotions, differing perspectives, and long-standing relationship dynamics. Even well-intentioned family members may clash over what's "best," especially when decisions involve safety, autonomy, finances, or end-of-life preferences. When cognitive decline—such as Alzheimer's or dementia—is involved, the emotional stakes are even higher. In these moments, effective guidance and compassionate mediation are crucial to preserving family unity and ensuring that care decisions remain centered on the dignity and well-being of the individual.

As a neutral, trusted professional, your elder law attorney offers families a safe and structured space to express concerns, clarify expectations, and align on goals. Their role is not to take sides, but to **facilitate respectful dialogue** and ensure that each voice is heard, especially the voice of the client, when possible. They help families move from conflict to clarity by identifying shared values, translating medical or legal information into everyday language, and guiding decision-making that reflects both clinical realities and personal priorities.

Elder law attorneys are often critical partners in this process. They help families **legally formalize care arrangements** by drafting powers of attorney, health care proxies, guardianship documents, and advance directives that ensure the elder's wishes are protected and upheld—even if they lose the ability to express them later. These legal documents are not only protective tools; they are also communication tools, helping families avoid future disagreements by clarifying responsibilities and establishing boundaries. When decisions must be made about long-term care placement, Medicaid eligibility, or asset protection, an elder law attorney can provide invaluable insight to prevent costly missteps.

In emotionally tense or legally complex cases, elder law attorneys can serve as a stabilizing force, working in tandem with care managers and financial advisors to ensure decisions are both ethically sound and legally secure. When multiple family members are involved, having legal clarity helps remove ambiguity and reduce friction. Care managers frequently collaborate with these professionals to ensure that the **care plan aligns with the legal plan**, so that the elder's voice is preserved across both personal care and financial decisions.

We encourage families to **shift from "winning" an argument to collaborating on a plan**. Emotions like guilt, fear, and grief often drive reactions, and by acknowledging these feelings with empathy, Elder law attorneys can help family members approach one another with understanding rather than judgment. Their guidance also includes defining roles, setting boundaries, and creating care agreements that prevent misunderstandings and reduce stress over time.

In the presence of long-distance relatives, blended family structures, or unresolved relational tension, my structured mediation process offers a path forward. Care plans developed with input from all stakeholders—guided by professional insight—lead to more peaceful transitions and healthier caregiving dynamics.

Ultimately, the goal is to restore the **focus back to the client**, ensuring that decisions made are not only medically appropriate but emotionally and ethically sound. When families work together with open hearts and clear guidance, care becomes more compassionate, sustainable, and aligned with what matters most.

Perhaps most importantly, having an elder law attorney on your team brings a deep sense of peace of mind. It's knowing that you're not facing difficult decisions alone—that someone with both compassion and legal expertise is walking beside you. Whether you're planning ahead or responding to a sudden need, this trusted ally provides clarity in moments of uncertainty and strength when advocacy is required. It's more than legal representation—it's the comfort of knowing your affairs are in order and your future is in capable hands.

# CHAPTER 19

# Essential Legal Documents
# for All Elderly Adults

### 1. Durable Power of Attorney (POA) for Finances

- Appoints a trusted individual to manage financial affairs if the elder becomes incapacitated.

- "Durable" means it remains in effect even if the person becomes mentally unable to make decisions.

### 2. Healthcare Power of Attorney (Health Care Proxy)

- Authorizes someone to make medical decisions on the elder's behalf when they are unable to do so.

- This person should understand the elder's values, medical preferences, and end-of-life wishes.

### 3. Advance Healthcare Directive (Living Will)

- Specifies what types of life-sustaining treatment the elder would or would not want (e.g., feeding tube, ventilator).

- Often works in conjunction with the healthcare POA.

### 4. HIPAA Authorization Form

- Grants permission for designated individuals to access the elder's medical information.

- Without this, even close family members can be restricted from important updates.

5. **Will**

   ○ Outlines how the elder's property and assets will be distributed after death.

   ○ Naming an executor ensures that someone they trust will carry out their wishes.

6. **Revocable Living Trust (when appropriate)**

   ○ Helps manage assets during life and distributes them after death without the need for probate.

   ○ Often recommended when there are significant assets, complex family dynamics, or blended families.

7. **Guardianship / Conservatorship Plan (as a last resort)**

   ○ If legal capacity has already been lost and no POA is in place, families may need to petition the court.

   ○ Planning ahead with POAs helps avoid this step.

8. **Beneficiary Designations Review**

   ○ Although not a document per se, reviewing and updating beneficiaries on life insurance, retirement accounts, and bank accounts is crucial.

   ○ These override a will if not properly aligned.

9. **Do Not Resuscitate (DNR) / POLST (Physician Orders for Life-Sustaining Treatment)**

   ○ A physician must sign medical orders and clearly communicated to emergency responders.

   ○ Often used in more advanced illness or hospice care settings.

## Why Having Documents In-Place Matters

Having these documents in place before a crisis allows elders to maintain control over their lives and decisions, ensures that trusted people are legally empowered to help them, and reduces emotional and financial stress for families. As care managers and dementia care specialists, we often work in tandem with elder law attorneys to make sure the **care plan aligns with the legal plan**, creating a safety net that honors the elder's wishes while protecting their health, dignity, and estate.

Find a reputable Elder Law Attorney and request a consultation. You'll be glad you did.

# CHAPTER 20

# Neurocognitive Exercises!

Neurocognitive exercise is essential because it helps keep the brain active, engaged, and functioning at its best—especially as we age. Just like physical exercise strengthens the body, mental activities such as puzzles, memory games, and problem-solving tasks help preserve and enhance cognitive abilities like memory, attention, and reasoning. But the true value of neurocognitive exercise isn't just about getting the "right" answers or finishing a task perfectly—it's about the process of thinking, learning, and challenging the brain. Each time we engage with a mental activity, we're building neural connections, improving mental flexibility, and giving our minds the workout they need to stay sharp.

It's important to remember that the journey matters more than the destination when it comes to brain health. Struggling with a math problem, searching for a hidden word, or finding the way through a maze—all of these actions activate and strengthen the brain, regardless of whether the final answer is correct. This shift in focus—from performance to participation—makes neurocognitive exercise more enjoyable and less stressful, encouraging consistency and long-term benefits. For seniors in particular, this approach can create a positive, rewarding experience that supports independence and quality of life.

**Let's get ready to exercise our brain and have fun doing it!**

# Word Search Puzzles

Word search puzzles are not only fun and relaxing, but they're also an excellent neurocognitive exercise that helps keep the brain active and healthy. As you scan for hidden words, your brain engages in pattern recognition, visual scanning, and sustained attention—all of which stimulate areas related to memory and focus. For seniors, especially, doing word searches regularly can support cognitive health by reinforcing vocabulary, improving concentration, and enhancing short-term memory. They offer a low-stress way to challenge the mind while providing a sense of accomplishment, making them both enjoyable and beneficial for maintaining mental sharpness

They help improve recognition by training the brain to quickly identify patterns, letters, and word structures within a complex visual field. As you search for specific words hidden among seemingly random letters, your brain practices distinguishing relevant information from distractions—a key aspect of visual recognition. This repeated process strengthens the brain's ability to scan and process visual data efficiently. For seniors, this is particularly valuable, as it helps maintain and even enhance the speed and accuracy of recognizing familiar words, names, and objects in daily life, such as reading labels, signs, or instructions. Over time, this sharpened recognition supports better reading comprehension and contributes to overall cognitive resilience.

# It's A Party!

| N | S | A | E | O | O | B | A | L | L | O | O | N | S |
|---|---|---|---|---|---|---|---|---|---|---|---|---|---|
| K | P | K | P | P | E | N | N | A | N | T | S | E | S |
| S | N | A | P | K | I | N | S | C | U | P | S | C | I |
| N | G | I | S | R | P | L | T | S | C | F | P | E | I |
| S | R | E | P | P | O | P | Y | T | R | A | C | N | P |
| E | C | E | O | A | C | A | K | E | N | C | I | T | E |
| T | A | N | S | P | O | O | N | S | G | T | R | E | C |
| A | N | N | R | P | O | E | O | N | T | S | I | R | R |
| L | D | F | E | U | N | O | T | E | O | R | B | P | E |
| P | L | O | N | N | E | P | F | E | F | E | B | I | A |
| C | E | R | N | C | E | N | F | N | F | W | O | E | M |
| T | S | K | A | H | O | L | L | C | I | O | N | C | H |
| B | P | S | B | C | I | A | A | N | S | L | S | E | F |
| G | I | F | T | S | F | A | L | O | O | F | T | S | B |

| | | |
|---|---|---|
| 1. Sign | 7. Centerpiece | 13. Party Poppers |
| 2. Confetti | 8. Plates | 14. Candles |
| 3. Ice cream | 9. Ribbons | 15. Napkins |
| 4. Pennant | 10. Cake | 16. Gifts |
| 5. Cups | 11. Flowers | 17. Punch |
| 6. Banner | 12. Balloons | 18. Forks |

# Flowers!

| | | | | | | | | | | | | |
|---|---|---|---|---|---|---|---|---|---|---|---|---|
| L | I | L | Y | C | D | D | F | B | D | E | L | B | O |
| Z | I | N | N | I | A | S | T | E | A | D | R | A | L |
| N | F | I | Q | V | N | U | R | G | F | U | O | B | N |
| N | D | N | T | X | L | N | S | O | F | L | B | Y | O |
| R | H | Y | C | I | O | F | X | N | O | M | N | S | I |
| Y | J | L | P | R | Y | L | Z | I | D | W | O | B | T |
| T | D | I | H | C | R | O | H | A | I | D | G | R | A |
| T | V | L | F | G | K | W | D | P | L | G | A | E | N |
| L | I | A | J | S | O | E | B | O | D | J | R | A | R |
| Y | O | L | O | N | Y | R | G | S | X | P | D | T | A |
| P | L | L | N | R | L | I | Y | S | N | A | P | H | C |
| P | E | A | U | O | R | M | T | C | V | O | A | O | Y |
| O | T | C | L | A | C | A | L | I | L | S | N | H | K |
| P | F | E | M | F | Y | S | I | A | D | E | S | T | V |

| | | |
|---|---|---|
| 1. Lily | 7. Poppy | 13. Tulip |
| 2. Zinnia | 8. Marigold | 14. Daisy |
| 3. Sunflower | 9. Calla Lily | 15. Pansy |
| 4. Begonia | 10. Orchid | 16. Violet |
| 5. Baby's Breath | 11. Daffodil | 17. Phlox |
| 6. Carnation | 12. Snapdragon | 18. Lilac |

# Travel!

| C | A | R | Y | C | D | D | F | B | D | E | L | B | L |
|---|---|---|---|---|---|---|---|---|---|---|---|---|---|
| Z | I | N | N | I | A | S | T | E | S | D | R | U | P |
| N | F | I | Q | V | N | U | R | G | F | U | G | B | L |
| I | L | N | T | X | L | N | S | O | F | G | B | Y | A |
| A | I | R | P | O | R | T | X | P | A | M | Y | S | E |
| R | G | L | P | R | U | L | Z | G | D | W | R | B | S |
| T | H | I | H | C | R | R | E | A | I | D | A | R | A |
| N | T | L | F | S | S | A | P | M | O | C | R | E | C |
| O | I | A | J | S | O | E | B | O | D | J | E | A | T |
| Y | O | L | E | D | I | S | T | E | K | C | I | T | I |
| R | L | L | N | R | L | I | Y | S | N | A | E | H | U |
| R | E | A | U | O | R | M | T | P | I | R | T | O | S |
| A | B | A | C | K | P | A | C | K | L | S | I | H | K |
| C | F | E | M | T | Y | T | R | O | P | S | S | A | P |

| | | |
|---|---|---|
| 1. Car | 7. Backpack | 13. Guide |
| 2. Plane | 8. Itinerary | 14. Map |
| 3. Passport | 9. Flight | 15. Compass |
| 4. Suitcase | 10. Train | 16. Trip |
| 5. Luggage | 11. Bus | 17. Airport |
| 6. Carryon | 12. Tour | 18. Tickets |

# Countries of the World!

| | | | | | | | | | | | | | |
|---|---|---|---|---|---|---|---|---|---|---|---|---|---|
| I | R | E | L | A | N | D | F | B | D | E | L | N | L |
| Z | I | D | N | A | L | G | N | E | S | D | R | I | P |
| D | F | I | Q | V | N | P | O | R | T | U | G | A | L |
| I | E | N | E | D | E | W | S | M | F | A | B | P | A |
| A | I | N | P | O | R | T | X | E | A | M | Y | S | E |
| R | U | L | M | R | U | L | Z | X | D | E | R | B | Y |
| A | H | S | H | A | R | R | E | I | I | R | A | R | L |
| N | N | L | T | S | R | A | P | C | O | I | R | E | A |
| O | I | I | J | R | O | K | B | O | D | C | E | A | T |
| N | O | L | H | D | A | A | D | A | N | A | C | E | I |
| A | L | L | N | C | L | G | R | E | E | C | E | R | U |
| P | E | A | A | N | I | T | N | E | G | R | A | O | S |
| A | B | C | R | O | A | T | I | A | L | S | I | K | K |
| J | F | E | M | T | Y | T | R | U | S | S | I | A | P |

| | | |
|---|---|---|
| 1. Ireland | 7. England | 13. Korea |
| 2. Russia | 8. Portugal | 14. America |
| 3. Italy | 9. Denmark | 15. Canada |
| 4. Australia | 10. China | 16. Argentina |
| 5. Croatia | 11. Japan | 17. Greece |
| 6. Spain | 12. Sweden | 18. Mexico |

# Grandma's House!

| A | P | R | O | N | D | D | F | B | D | E | L | H | L |
|---|---|---|---|---|---|---|---|---|---|---|---|---|---|
| Z | X | O | B | G | N | I | W | E | S | D | L | A | P |
| N | F | D | S | V | N | U | R | L | F | U | E | I | L |
| I | L | E | T | R | L | N | E | O | F | G | B | R | K |
| A | I | N | O | R | O | L | L | E | R | S | R | N | O |
| H | G | T | P | R | R | T | P | G | D | W | E | E | O |
| S | H | U | H | L | R | H | A | A | I | D | N | T | B |
| I | T | R | N | S | O | A | N | L | O | C | N | E | T |
| D | I | E | J | S | E | E | S | O | O | J | I | A | E |
| Y | I | S | E | L | O | T | I | O | N | C | D | T | K |
| D | L | L | B | R | L | I | Y | S | N | A | R | H | C |
| N | E | I | U | O | E | D | I | U | G | V | T | E | O |
| A | B | A | T | H | T | U | B | N | R | U | A | H | P |
| C | F | E | O | I | D | A | R | O | P | N | O | R | I |

| | | |
|---|---|---|
| 1. Apron | 7. Hair Net | 13. TV Guide |
| 2. Sewing Box | 8. Pocketbook | 14. Dentures |
| 3. Candy Dish | 9. Radio | 15. Lotion |
| 4. Iron | 10. Dinner Bell | 16. Percolator |
| 5. Bathtub | 11. Pans | 17. Rollers |
| 6. Bible | 12. Pots | 18. Hose |

# United States of America!

| N | A | R | Y | C | D | A | I | G | R | O | E | G | M |
|---|---|---|---|---|---|---|---|---|---|---|---|---|---|
| Z | E | N | N | I | A | S | A | S | N | A | K | R | A |
| N | E | W | Q | V | N | U | R | S | F | U | G | B | I |
| I | L | R | J | X | L | N | S | A | F | G | B | Y | N |
| A | R | R | A | E | R | T | X | X | A | M | A | S | E |
| M | O | L | N | W | R | L | Z | E | D | W | I | F | S |
| I | C | I | O | C | A | S | E | T | I | D | N | L | A |
| C | I | L | Z | S | S | L | E | M | I | H | I | O | C |
| H | X | A | I | S | A | E | E | Y | I | J | G | R | T |
| I | E | L | R | D | I | S | T | D | A | C | R | I | I |
| G | M | L | A | R | L | I | Y | X | W | A | I | D | A |
| A | W | V | E | R | M | O | N | T | A | R | V | A | W |
| N | E | W | Y | O | R | K | C | E | H | S | I | E | O |
| N | N | E | M | T | Y | T | A | N | A | I | D | N | I |

| | | |
|---|---|---|
| 1. Ohio | 7. Iowa | 13. Hawaii |
| 2. Michigan | 8. Nevada | 14. Arkansas |
| 3. Indiana | 9. New Mexico | 15. Georgia |
| 4. New York | 10. Arizona | 16. Vermont |
| 5. New Jersey | 11. Maine | 17. Texas |
| 6. Florida | 12. Delaware | 18. Virginia |

# Colors!

| W | A | E | Y | C | D | D | F | B | E | U | L | B | L |
|---|---|---|---|---|---|---|---|---|---|---|---|---|---|
| H | I | U | N | I | W | O | L | L | E | Y | R | R | P |
| I | F | L | Q | V | N | U | N | A | T | U | G | O | L |
| T | L | B | T | X | L | N | S | C | F | G | B | W | A |
| E | I | Y | I | V | O | R | Y | K | A | M | Y | N | E |
| R | G | K | P | U | R | P | L | E | A | W | R | B | E |
| T | R | S | H | C | R | R | E | A | I | U | E | R | S |
| N | E | L | F | S | S | T | P | M | O | I | Q | E | I |
| P | E | A | C | H | E | E | B | O | G | J | E | A | O |
| Y | N | L | E | L | I | S | T | E | K | C | I | T | U |
| R | L | L | O | R | A | N | G | E | N | A | E | H | Q |
| R | E | I | U | O | R | M | T | P | I | R | T | D | R |
| M | V | A | C | K | P | A | C | K | L | S | I | E | U |
| C | O | G | I | D | N | I | R | O | P | S | S | R | T |

1. Green
2. Blue
3. Red
4. Indigo
5. Violet
6. Orange
7. Black
8. White
9. Peach
10. Purple
11. Tan
12. Turquoise
13. Aqua
14. Sky Blue
15. Ivory
16. Brown
17. Beige
18. Yellow

# Tools in the Garage!

| L | A | R | E | R | A | U | Q | S | T | E | L | B | W |
|---|---|---|---|---|---|---|---|---|---|---|---|---|---|
| Z | A | N | R | I | A | S | N | A | I | L | S | U | A |
| N | F | D | Q | R | N | U | R | G | F | E | R | B | S |
| W | A | S | D | X | W | N | S | O | F | V | E | Y | H |
| A | I | S | P | E | R | O | X | P | A | E | I | S | E |
| V | I | C | E | R | R | L | M | G | N | L | L | B | R |
| T | H | R | H | C | A | I | R | P | U | M | P | J | A |
| N | T | E | F | S | K | A | P | M | T | C | R | A | C |
| R | I | W | J | S | E | E | S | O | S | J | E | C | T |
| E | O | S | E | D | I | T | T | E | K | C | I | K | I |
| M | L | L | N | R | L | I | T | E | H | C | T | A | R |
| M | E | A | U | O | R | M | T | P | I | R | T | O | S |
| A | B | A | B | K | P | A | C | K | L | S | I | H | K |
| H | F | E | R | E | V | I | R | D | W | E | R | C | S |

| | | |
|---|---|---|
| 1. Screwdriver | 7. Saw | 13. Nuts |
| 2. Hammer | 8. Vice | 14. Bolts |
| 3. Jack | 9. Pliers | 15. Washer |
| 4. Ladder | 10. Nails | 16. Ratchet |
| 5. Rake | 11. Screws | 17. T-Square |
| 6. Air Pump | 12. Level | 18. Mower |

# Cakes & Pies!

| C | H | E | R | R | Y | Y | R | E | B | E | U | L | B |
|---|---|---|---|---|---|---|---|---|---|---|---|---|---|
| Z | I | E | N | I | A | S | T | E | S | D | R | U | P |
| O | T | I | M | V | P | E | A | C | H | U | G | P | E |
| T | L | U | T | I | P | N | E | O | F | D | B | U | C |
| A | I | E | N | O | L | T | L | P | A | R | Y | M | A |
| T | G | L | M | O | E | Y | T | G | D | A | R | P | N |
| O | H | I | H | O | C | R | E | A | I | T | R | K | A |
| P | T | L | F | S | N | O | U | K | O | S | E | I | C |
| T | I | A | J | S | O | E | T | O | D | U | B | N | E |
| E | O | E | T | A | L | O | C | O | H | C | W | T | I |
| E | S | U | G | A | R | C | R | E | A | M | A | H | P |
| W | E | A | U | O | B | R | A | B | U | H | R | O | T |
| S | B | A | C | K | P | A | C | K | L | S | T | H | O |
| B | L | A | C | K | B | E | R | R | Y | S | S | A | P |

| | | |
|---|---|---|
| 1. Cherry | 7. Rhubarb | 13. Custard |
| 2. Apple | 8. Blackberry | 14. Sugar Cream |
| 3. Blueberry | 9. Pecan | 15. Coconut |
| 4. Strawberry | 10. Pumpkin | 16. Turtle |
| 5. Peach | 11. Sweet Potato | 17. Potpie |
| 6. Lemon | 12. Chocolate | 18. Key Lime |

# At the Doctor's Office!

| S | T | E | T | H | O | S | C | O | P | E | L | T | L |
|---|---|---|---|---|---|---|---|---|---|---|---|---|---|
| R | I | E | Z | I | T | I | N | A | S | D | R | H | S |
| N | F | I | Q | V | N | U | R | G | F | U | G | E | S |
| L | L | N | T | X | L | T | H | G | I | L | B | R | E |
| L | P | U | L | S | E | O | X | P | O | M | S | M | R |
| A | S | E | L | D | E | E | N | V | P | W | R | O | P |
| B | H | K | H | C | E | R | E | I | I | D | E | M | E |
| N | T | G | F | S | G | S | T | M | S | C | Z | E | D |
| O | I | A | J | S | A | Q | B | S | E | J | E | T | F |
| T | O | L | E | D | D | S | T | L | P | C | E | E | F |
| T | A | B | L | E | N | I | Y | U | I | A | W | R | U |
| O | E | A | U | O | A | E | U | S | W | I | T | O | C |
| C | B | A | C | K | B | S | S | P | R | A | H | S | P |
| C | F | E | M | M | O | O | R | M | A | X | E | A | B |

1. Stethoscope
2. BPCuff
3. Exam Room
4. Cotton Ball
5. Table
6. Bandage
7. Qtip
8. Sanitizer
9. Gloves
10. Sharps
11. Thermometer
12. Pulse Ox
13. Tweezers
14. Tissue
15. Needles
16. Wipes
17. Light
8. EKG

# Hats!

| C | A | R | B | C | D | D | E | I | N | O | O | B | L |
|---|---|---|---|---|---|---|---|---|---|---|---|---|---|
| Z | I | P | O | R | K | P | I | E | S | D | R | N | P |
| B | P | I | H | V | N | F | R | G | T | V | G | E | L |
| E | F | A | O | X | L | E | S | O | A | I | B | W | A |
| A | I | L | N | O | Y | D | X | P | H | S | Y | S | E |
| N | G | L | A | A | U | O | Z | G | P | O | R | B | S |
| I | H | I | H | T | M | R | B | A | O | R | A | O | A |
| E | T | L | F | S | S | A | O | W | T | C | Y | Y | C |
| O | I | T | J | S | W | O | W | O | O | J | B | A | T |
| Y | B | E | R | E | T | S | L | E | K | C | L | T | E |
| R | L | M | N | R | L | I | E | S | N | A | I | H | K |
| R | Z | L | U | O | R | M | R | P | I | R | R | O | C |
| A | E | E | C | P | A | C | T | A | L | F | T | H | U |
| C | F | H | P | A | C | L | L | A | B | E | S | A | B |

| | | |
|---|---|---|
| 1. Baseball Cap | 7. Bucket | 13. Pork Pie |
| 2. Helmet | 8. Boonie | 14. Trilby |
| 3. Beret | 9. Panama | 15. Top Hat |
| 4. Cowboy | 10. Fez | 16. Boho |
| 5. Fedora | 11. Newsboy | 17. Flat Cap |
| 6. Beanie | 12. Bowler | 18. Visor |

# Cars!

| C | A | R | Y | C | D | D | F | B | D | F | L | B | M |
|---|---|---|---|---|---|---|---|---|---|---|---|---|---|
| H | I | A | T | O | Y | O | T | E | O | D | R | M | E |
| E | F | H | Q | V | N | U | R | R | F | U | G | W | R |
| V | L | O | T | X | L | N | D | O | F | G | B | Y | C |
| Y | I | N | P | O | C | A | L | L | I | D | A | C | D |
| R | G | D | P | R | I | I | Z | G | D | W | R | B | E |
| T | H | A | H | D | A | R | E | A | I | D | A | R | S |
| N | T | L | U | D | S | A | N | A | V | I | N | I | M |
| O | I | A | N | S | E | D | A | N | E | G | D | O | D |
| Y | S | U | B | A | R | U | T | E | A | C | I | T | I |
| R | Y | L | N | R | L | I | Y | S | N | S | E | H | U |
| H | E | A | D | Z | A | M | T | D | I | R | S | A | S |
| A | B | U | I | C | K | A | C | L | L | S | I | I | K |
| C | F | E | M | T | Y | T | R | O | P | S | S | K | N |

| | | |
|---|---|---|
| 1. Buick | 7. Nissan | 13. Kia |
| 2. Olds | 8. Toyota | 14. Honda |
| 3. Chevy | 9. Mercedes | 15. Sedan |
| 4. Dodge | 10. BMW | 16. Cadillac |
| 5. Ford | 11. Hyundai | 17. Audi |
| 6. Mazda | 12. Mini Van | 18. Subaru |

# In a Restaurant!

| T | A | B | L | E | S | M | F | B | D | E | L | B | S |
|---|---|---|---|---|---|---|---|---|---|---|---|---|---|
| Z | I | N | N | I | E | S | T | E | S | D | R | U | I |
| N | F | I | Q | N | N | U | S | R | I | A | H | C | L |
| I | L | N | U | X | L | N | E | N | F | S | B | Y | V |
| A | I | E | P | O | T | S | E | P | Y | M | Y | S | E |
| R | S | L | A | R | C | H | Z | A | D | W | K | B | R |
| T | S | I | N | T | C | R | R | A | I | I | A | R | W |
| S | T | L | S | T | S | T | P | M | L | R | R | E | A |
| R | O | K | I | S | O | S | B | L | D | J | E | A | R |
| E | B | K | E | D | F | S | E | S | G | N | O | T | E |
| V | S | L | N | E | L | T | Y | S | N | A | E | H | U |
| R | U | A | H | O | R | M | A | N | A | G | E | R | S |
| E | B | C | O | O | K | S | C | K | L | S | I | H | K |
| S | F | E | M | T | Y | T | R | S | T | S | E | U | G |

| | | |
|---|---|---|
| 1. Tables | 7. Busboys | 13. Pots |
| 2. Chairs | 8. Chefs | 14. Pans |
| 3. Menus | 9. Cooks | 15. Skillets |
| 4. Silverware | 10. Manager | 16. Spatulas |
| 5. Guests | 11. Kitchen | 17. Tongs |
| 6. Servers | 12. Bar | 18. Serving Trays |

# Farm Animals!

| C | O | W | Y | C | D | O | N | K | E | Y | L | B | L |
|---|---|---|---|---|---|---|---|---|---|---|---|---|---|
| Z | I | N | N | H | A | S | T | E | S | D | R | U | P |
| N | F | I | Q | I | N | U | U | G | F | L | L | U | B |
| I | K | N | T | C | L | N | R | O | F | G | B | Y | E |
| A | C | R | P | K | R | S | Y | E | K | R | U | T | E |
| M | U | L | E | E | U | L | E | G | D | W | R | B | S |
| T | D | I | H | N | R | S | Y | A | I | D | T | A | C |
| N | T | L | F | S | O | T | I | B | B | A | R | E | C |
| O | I | A | J | O | O | E | B | O | D | J | E | E | T |
| Y | O | L | G | D | I | S | T | T | K | C | I | S | I |
| H | E | N | S | R | L | L | A | M | A | A | E | R | U |
| R | E | G | U | O | A | M | T | P | I | O | T | O | S |
| A | I | A | C | K | M | A | C | K | L | S | G | H | K |
| P | F | E | M | T | B | T | R | O | O | S | T | E | R |

| | | |
|---|---|---|
| 1. Cow | 7. Donkey | 13. Rabbit |
| 2. Chicken | 8. Mule | 14. Goose |
| 3. Pig | 9. Goat | 15. Duck |
| 4. Horse | 10. Lamb | 16. Turkey |
| 5. Hens | 11. Cat | 17. Bees |
| 6. Rooster | 12. Bull | 18. Llama |

# Zoo Animals!

| C | A | R | Y | C | D | D | D | R | A | P | O | E | L |
|---|---|---|---|---|---|---|---|---|---|---|---|---|---|
| H | I | N | N | R | E | D | I | P | S | O | R | I | P |
| E | P | E | N | G | U | I | N | S | F | L | G | M | L |
| E | L | R | O | T | A | G | I | L | L | A | B | P | A |
| T | T | R | P | O | R | T | X | P | E | R | Y | A | E |
| A | U | L | P | B | U | L | Z | K | D | B | R | L | S |
| H | R | E | L | E | P | H | A | N | T | E | A | A | A |
| N | T | F | F | A | S | N | P | M | O | A | R | E | C |
| O | L | F | Y | V | S | E | I | B | I | R | D | S | T |
| Y | E | A | E | E | I | S | T | E | K | C | I | T | I |
| R | L | R | K | R | L | I | Y | S | N | A | E | H | G |
| R | E | I | N | O | R | M | S | R | E | T | T | O | E |
| A | B | G | O | R | I | L | L | A | L | S | I | H | R |
| C | F | E | M | T | Y | T | R | O | P | N | O | I | L |

| | | |
|---|---|---|
| 1. Lion | 7. Giraffe | 13. Alligator |
| 2. Tiger | 8. Elephant | 14. Turtle |
| 3. Leopard | 9. Otters | 15. Snake |
| 4. Cheetah | 10. Penguin | 16. Spider |
| 5. Monkey | 11. Polar Bear | 17. Impala |
| 6. Gorilla | 12. Birds | 18. Beaver |

# Life Under the Sea!

| C | S | H | A | R | K | D | R | E | T | S | B | O | L |
|---|---|---|---|---|---|---|---|---|---|---|---|---|---|
| Z | E | N | N | N | I | H | P | L | O | D | R | U | P |
| N | A | S | W | O | R | D | F | I | S | H | G | B | L |
| I | H | E | T | X | L | N | S | O | F | G | W | Y | A |
| A | O | A | P | O | R | E | X | P | A | M | H | S | E |
| R | R | W | P | R | E | L | T | R | U | T | A | E | S |
| T | S | E | H | C | R | R | S | E | I | D | L | R | A |
| N | E | E | F | S | S | A | S | E | O | C | E | E | N |
| O | I | D | B | S | O | E | A | F | D | J | E | O | T |
| Y | O | B | E | D | R | S | L | E | K | C | I | T | I |
| R | O | L | N | R | E | I | G | S | P | L | E | H | H |
| L | E | A | U | O | T | M | A | P | A | I | T | O | S |
| A | S | A | C | K | A | A | E | E | L | S | H | H | I |
| C | O | R | A | L | W | T | S | O | P | S | S | S | F |

| | | |
|---|---|---|
| 1. Fish | 7. Dolphin | 13. Ship |
| 2. Coral | 8. Sea Turtle | 14. Reef |
| 3. Water | 9. Sea Weed | 15. Sea Glass |
| 4. Sea Horse | 10. Sword Fish | 16. Sea Lion |
| 5. Shark | 11. Eel | 17. Shrimp |
| 6. Whale | 12. Sand | 18. Lobster |

# At the Office!

| C | A | R | Y | C | N | O | I | T | P | E | C | E | R |
|---|---|---|---|---|---|---|---|---|---|---|---|---|---|
| O | W | H | I | T | E | B | O | A | R | D | R | B | P |
| M | F | A | X | V | N | U | R | G | F | P | M | A | L |
| P | L | P | T | E | L | H | S | O | E | G | O | T | A |
| U | I | A | E | O | N | C | X | N | A | M | O | H | S |
| T | G | P | L | R | U | N | S | G | D | W | R | R | N |
| E | H | E | E | C | S | U | H | A | I | D | H | O | E |
| R | T | R | P | S | L | P | R | P | O | C | C | O | T |
| R | I | A | H | S | I | E | B | E | E | J | N | M | I |
| I | O | L | O | E | C | L | T | E | T | L | U | S | L |
| A | L | L | N | L | N | O | Y | S | K | N | L | H | L |
| H | E | A | E | B | E | H | T | P | I | N | I | T | U |
| C | B | A | C | A | P | A | C | K | L | S | I | R | B |
| D | E | S | K | T | R | E | L | P | A | T | S | A | P |

| | | |
|---|---|---|
| 1. Desk | 7. Reception | 13. Telephone |
| 2. Chair | 8. Pencils | 14. Fax |
| 3. Table | 9. Whiteboard | 15. Paper |
| 4. Stapler | 10. Bullitens | 16. Ink |
| 5. Computer | 11. Lunchroom | 17. Holepunch |
| 6. Printer | 12. Bathrooms | 18. Pens |

# Around the House!

| | | | | | | | | | | | | | |
|---|---|---|---|---|---|---|---|---|---|---|---|---|---|
| E | A | B | Y | C | D | D | F | R | E | W | O | H | S |
| L | I | A | N | I | A | R | E | T | U | P | M | O | C |
| P | F | T | Q | V | N | R | R | G | F | S | G | B | L |
| O | L | H | T | X | L | N | E | O | N | G | B | Y | A |
| E | I | T | P | O | R | T | K | I | A | R | U | G | S |
| P | G | U | P | R | S | L | A | G | D | W | R | B | S |
| T | H | B | H | T | R | T | M | A | I | D | A | R | A |
| N | N | L | E | S | R | A | E | D | O | M | M | O | C |
| O | A | P | J | U | O | E | E | O | S | J | E | A | T |
| Y | M | L | C | D | I | S | F | E | P | D | I | T | I |
| T | O | A | S | T | E | R | F | S | M | A | E | H | U |
| V | T | A | U | O | R | M | O | P | A | R | T | B | S |
| A | T | A | B | L | E | S | C | K | L | S | I | B | K |
| C | O | U | C | H | Y | R | E | N | I | L | C | E | R |

| | | |
|---|---|---|
| 1. Couch | 7. Coffee Maker | 13. Pets |
| 2. TV | 8. Toaster | 14. People |
| 3. Recliner | 9. Beds | 15. Car |
| 4. Ottoman | 10. Commode | 16. Computer |
| 5. Lamps | 11. Shower | 17. Rugs |
| 6. Tables | 12. Bathtub | 18. Curtains |

# Musical Instruments!

| C | A | R | Y | C | D | D | T | E | P | M | U | R | T |
|---|---|---|---|---|---|---|---|---|---|---|---|---|---|
| T | R | O | M | B | O | N | E | E | S | D | R | U | M |
| N | F | I | Q | V | N | U | R | G | F | U | G | B | L |
| I | R | U | P | R | I | G | H | T | B | A | S | S | A |
| A | E | R | V | I | O | L | A | P | N | A | G | R | O |
| T | N | L | I | R | N | A | G | R | O | W | R | B | E |
| E | C | I | O | H | R | R | E | O | I | N | A | R | N |
| N | H | L | L | S | A | A | P | M | L | C | A | E | O |
| I | H | A | I | A | O | R | B | O | E | L | E | I | H |
| R | O | L | N | D | I | S | P | E | B | O | E | T | P |
| A | R | L | N | R | L | R | Y | S | E | A | B | C | O |
| L | N | A | T | R | I | A | N | G | L | E | T | O | X |
| C | B | L | A | B | M | Y | C | K | L | S | I | H | A |
| F | L | U | T | E | Y | T | R | O | S | S | S | A | S |

| | | |
|---|---|---|
| 1. Flute | 7. Cymbal | 13. Upright Bass |
| 2. Clarinet | 8. Bells | 14. Cello |
| 3. Trumpet | 9. Triangle | 15. Violin |
| 4. Trombone | 10. Oboe | 16. Viola |
| 5. French Horn | 11. Saxophone | 17. Harp |
| 6. Drum | 12. Piano | 18. Organ |

# Fruits!

| C | P | B | Y | Y | R | R | E | B | W | A | R | T | S |
|---|---|---|---|---|---|---|---|---|---|---|---|---|---|
| Z | I | L | N | I | A | S | T | E | S | M | U | L | P |
| N | N | A | Q | V | N | E | R | G | F | A | G | B | Y |
| I | E | C | T | N | L | P | A | O | F | N | B | Y | R |
| A | A | K | P | O | R | O | X | N | A | G | Y | S | R |
| R | P | B | E | M | I | L | Z | G | A | O | R | B | E |
| T | P | E | H | E | R | A | E | A | I | N | A | R | B |
| N | L | R | F | L | S | N | P | M | O | C | A | E | E |
| D | E | R | E | G | N | A | R | O | D | J | E | B | U |
| U | O | Y | E | D | I | C | T | E | K | P | I | T | L |
| R | L | L | N | R | L | I | Y | S | N | A | E | H | B |
| I | E | A | U | O | E | L | P | P | A | R | G | A | S |
| A | Y | A | P | A | P | A | C | K | I | W | I | I | R |
| N | F | E | M | T | Y | T | O | C | I | R | P | A | F |

| 1. Apple | 7. Blackberry | 13. Mango |
|----------|---------------|-----------|
| 2. Orange | 8. Strawberry | 14. Papaya |
| 3. Lemon | 9. Banana | 15. Pineapple |
| 4. Lime | 10. Kiwi | 16. Durian |
| 5. Blueberry | 11. Plum | 17. Apricot |
| 6. Canalope | 12. Pear | 18. Fig |

# Maze Puzzles

Maze puzzles are fun and engaging activities that offer seniors an enjoyable way to challenge their minds while providing a satisfying sense of accomplishment. Navigating through a maze requires focus, patience, and strategy, all of which turn the puzzle into a mentally stimulating experience rather than just a pastime. The visual search for the correct path activates spatial awareness and planning skills, and the trial-and-error nature of mazes encourages problem-solving and persistence. Because mazes are both simple to start and rewarding to complete, they strike a great balance between mental challenge and entertainment, making them especially appealing for older adults looking to stay mentally active.

Beyond entertainment, maze puzzles offer significant neurocognitive benefits that support everyday functioning. Working through a maze strengthens spatial reasoning, hand-eye coordination, and executive functioning—the brain's ability to plan, shift focus, and make decisions. These skills are directly related to daily activities such as navigating a new environment, remembering directions, organizing tasks, or even safely maneuvering through crowded places. By exercising these mental faculties in a fun, low-pressure way, seniors can enhance their cognitive resilience, which helps maintain independence and confidence in managing everyday life.

**Start**

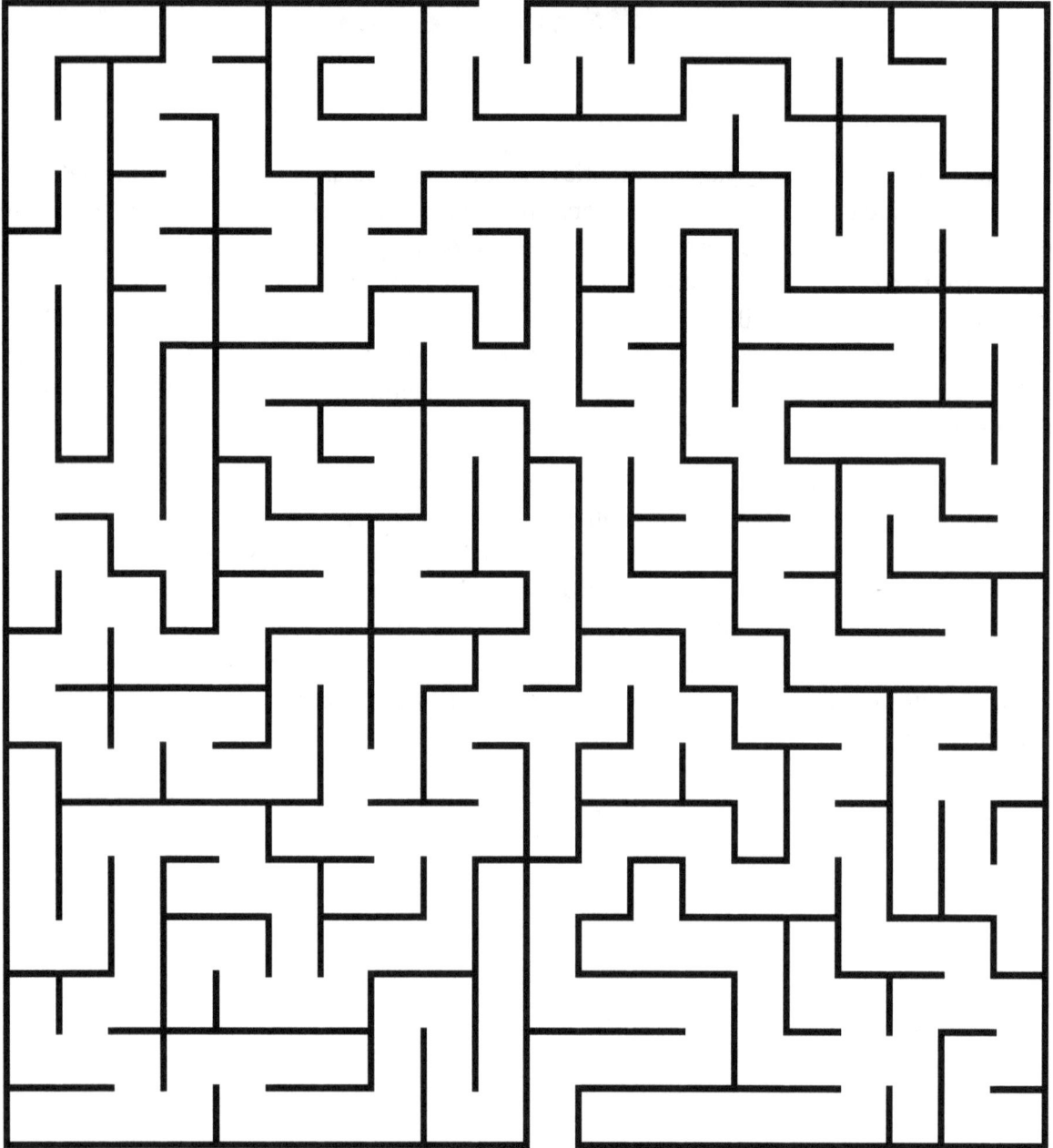

**Finish**

82

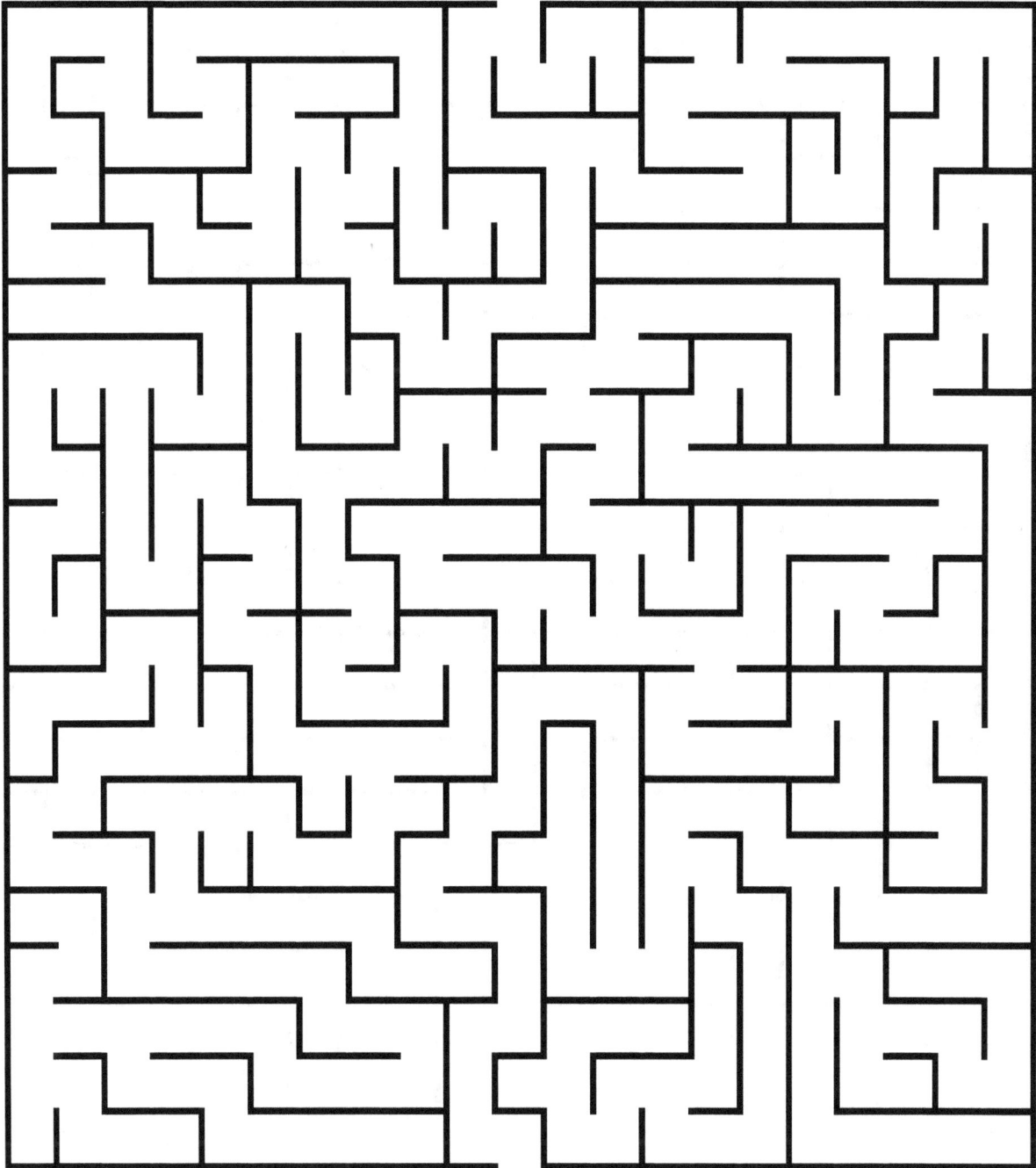

Finish

Start

Finish

84

**Start**

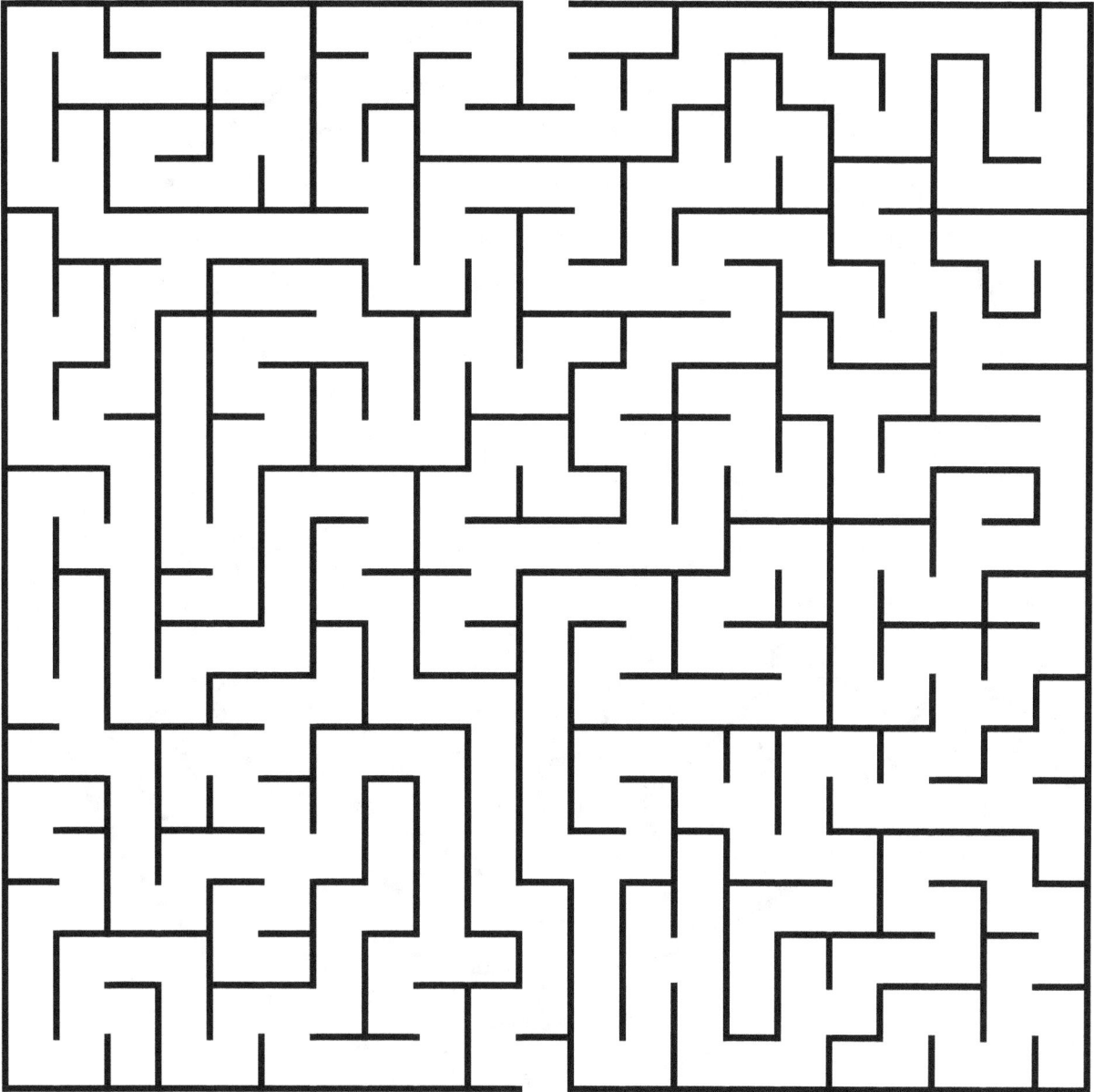

**Finish**

85

**Start**

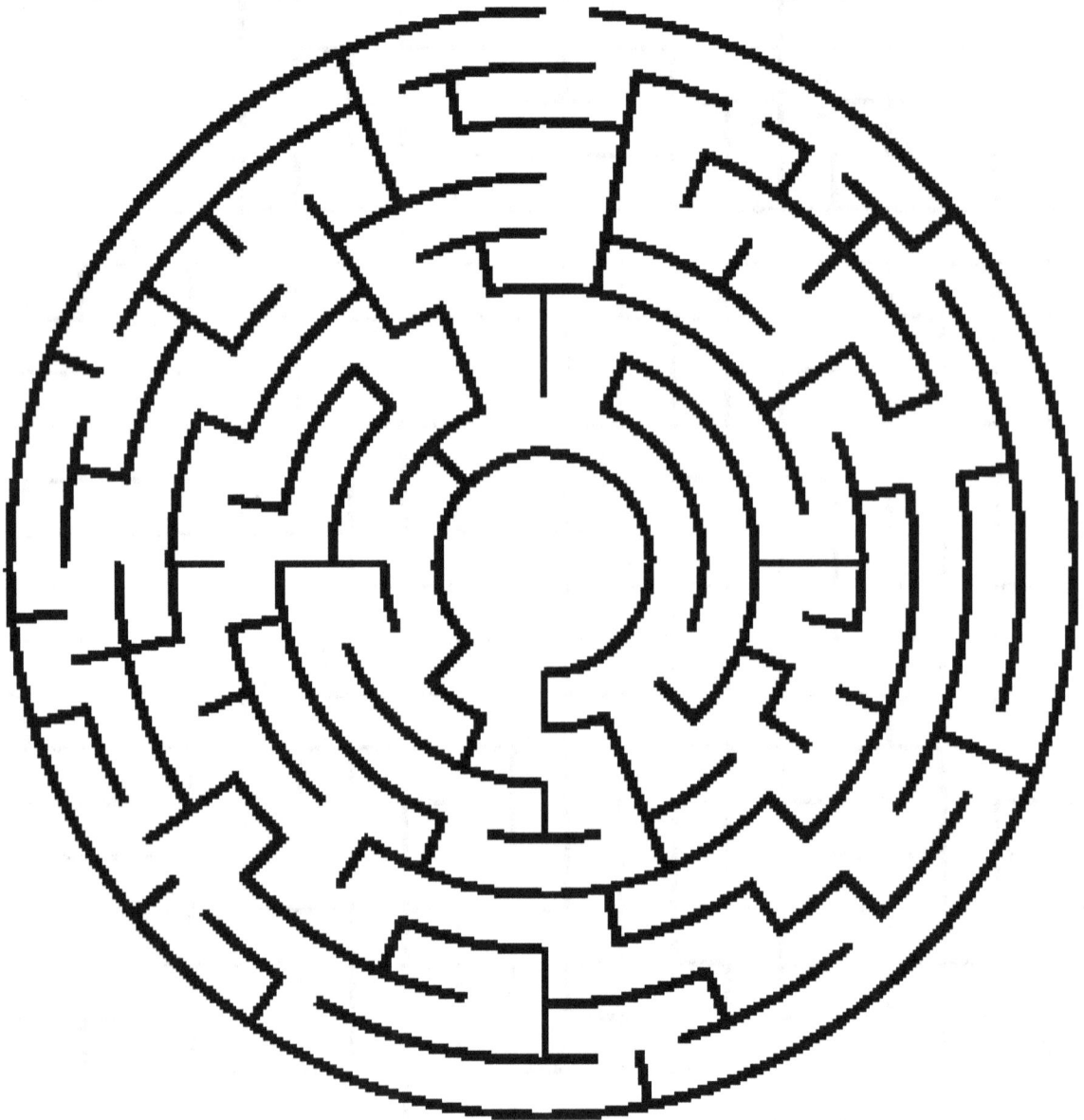

**Finish in the center.**

**Start**

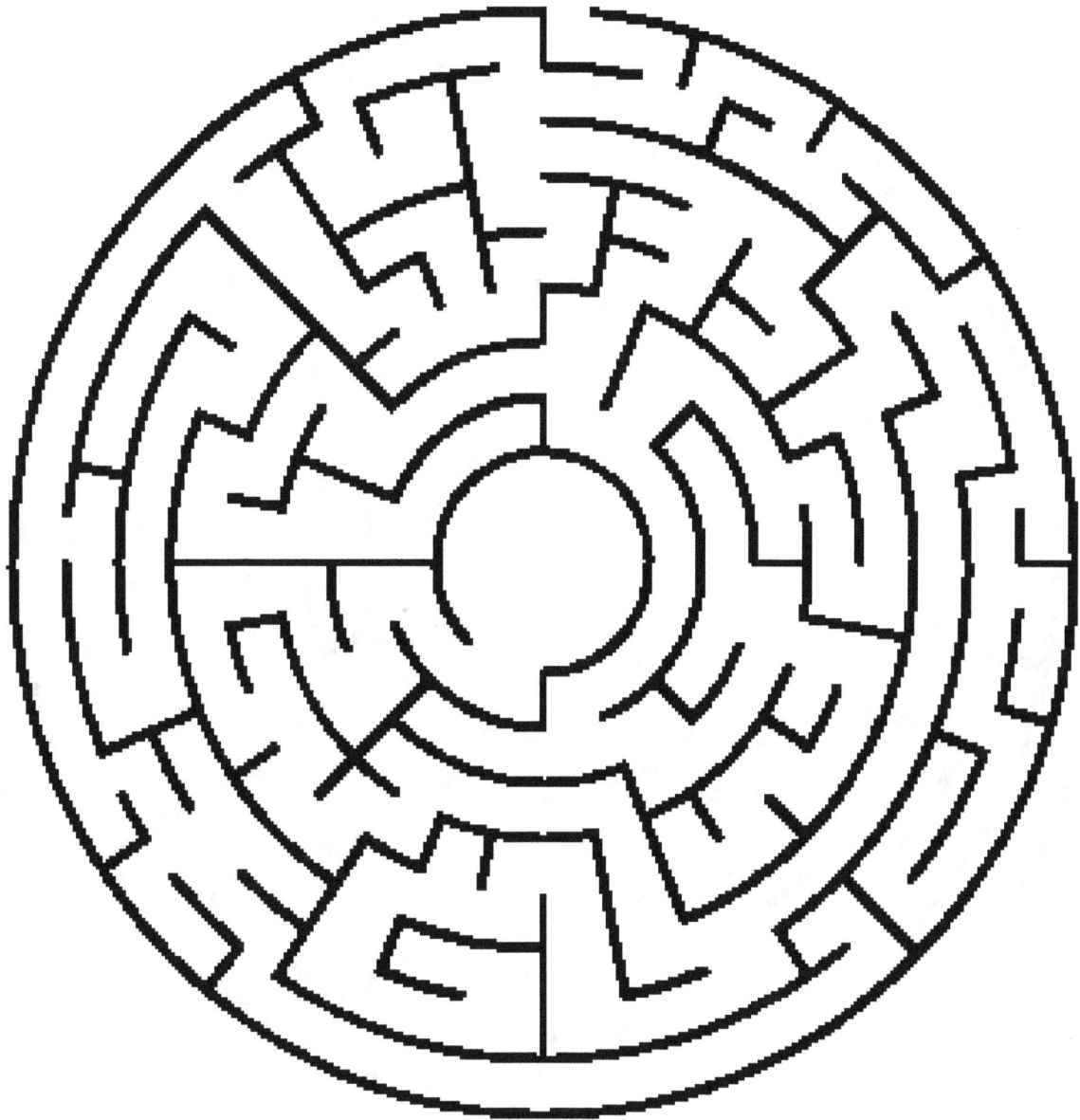

**Finish in the center.**

**Start**

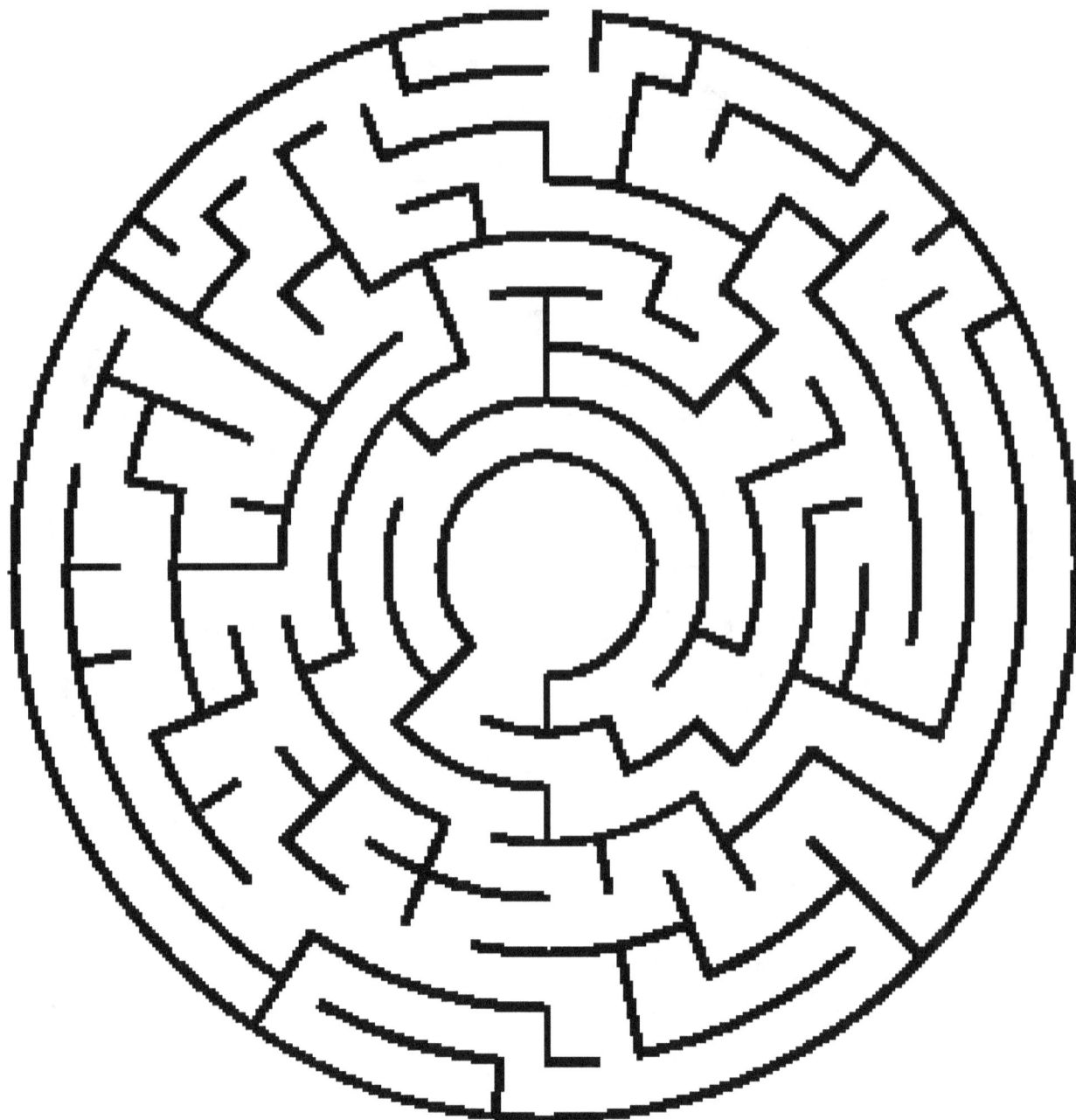

**Finish in the center.**

**Start**

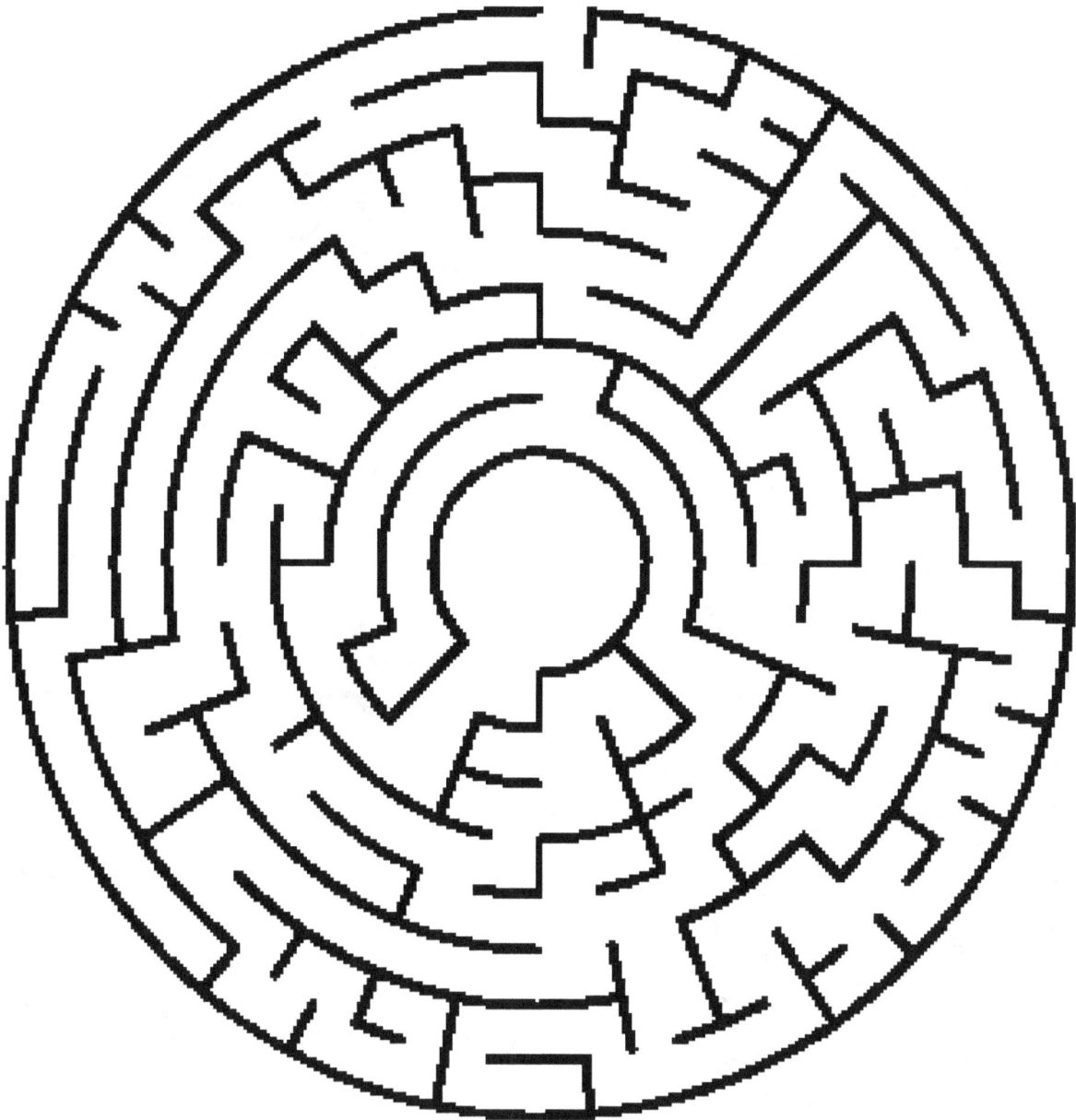

**Finish in the center.**

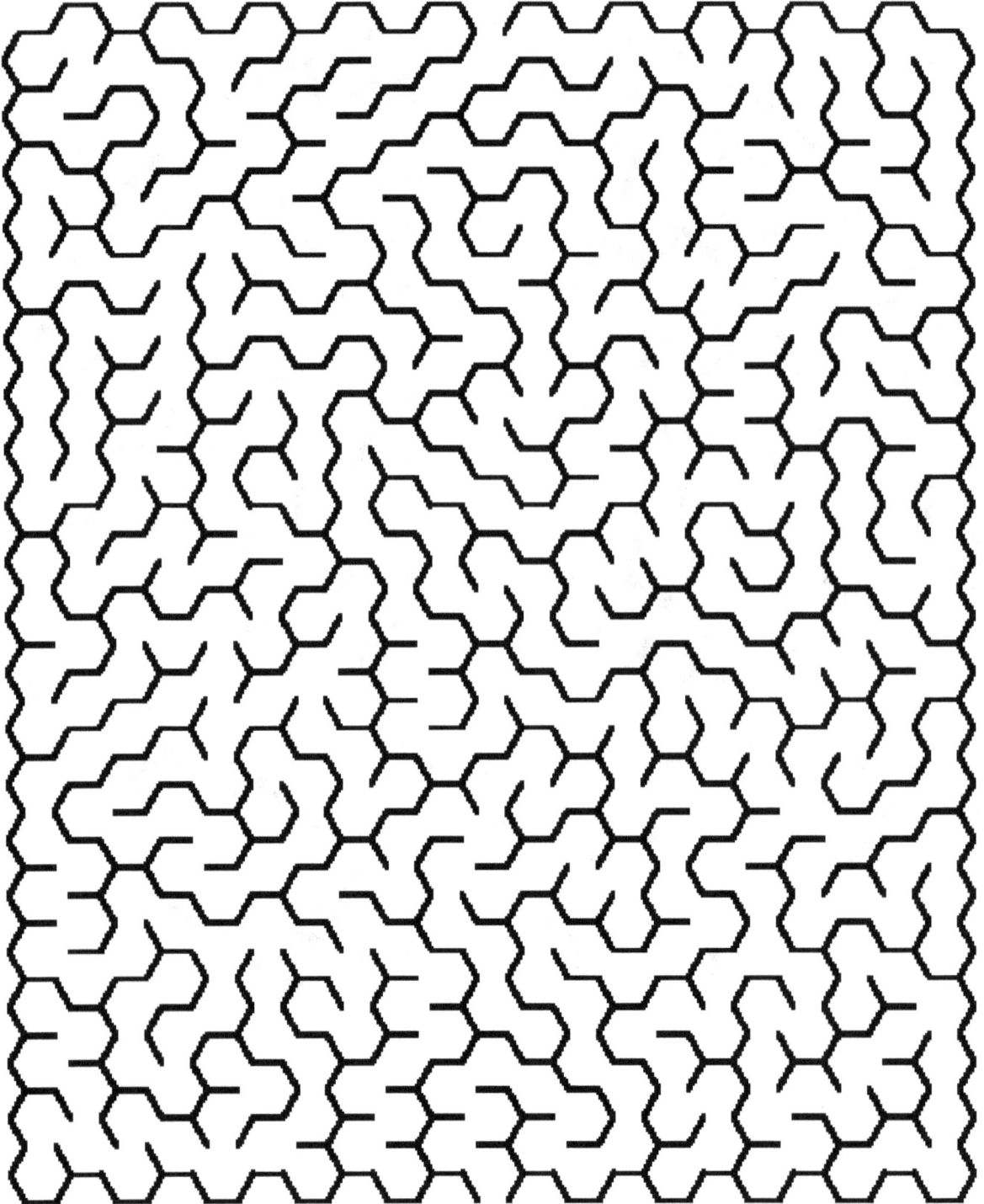

**Start**

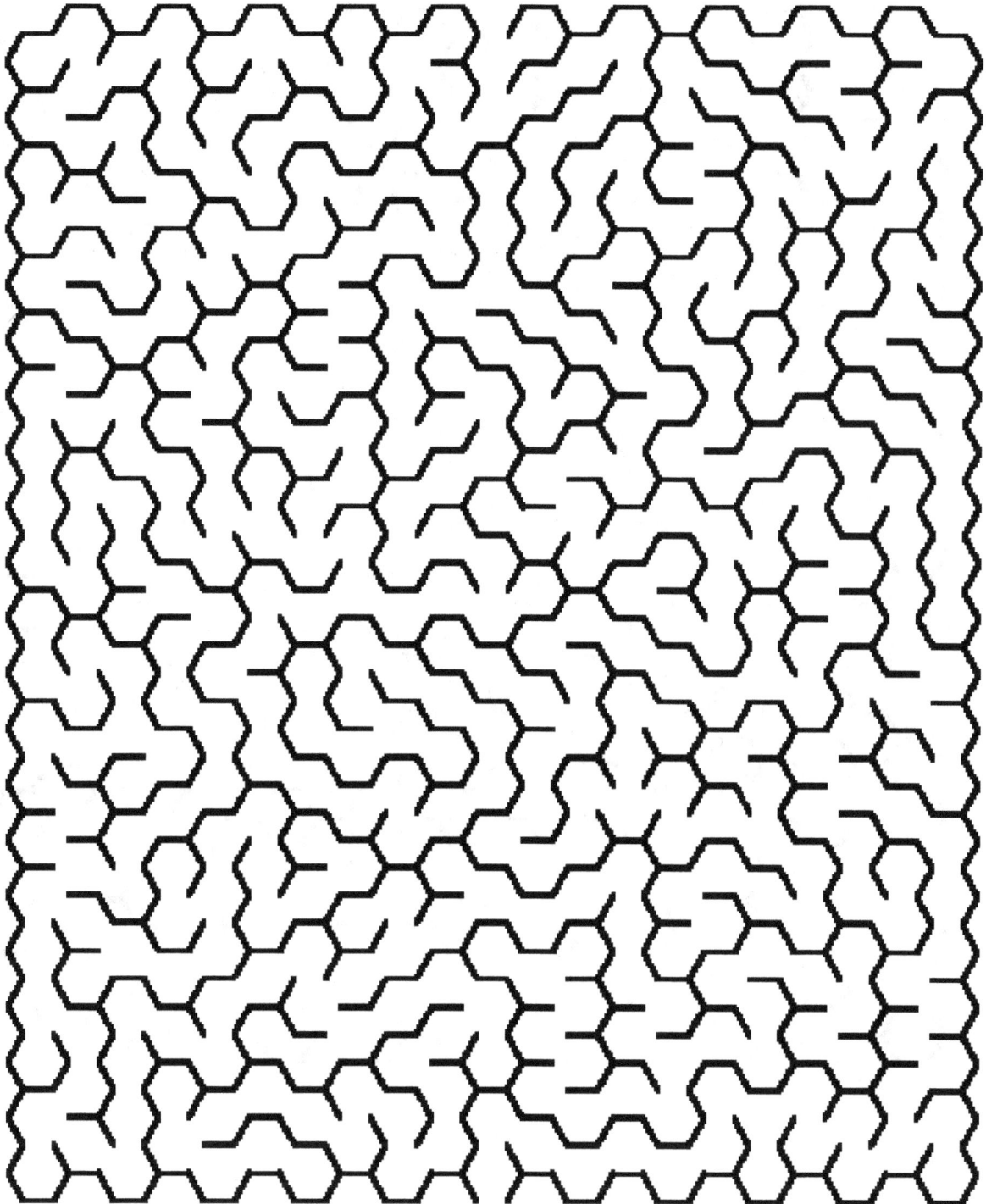

**Finish**

91

Finish

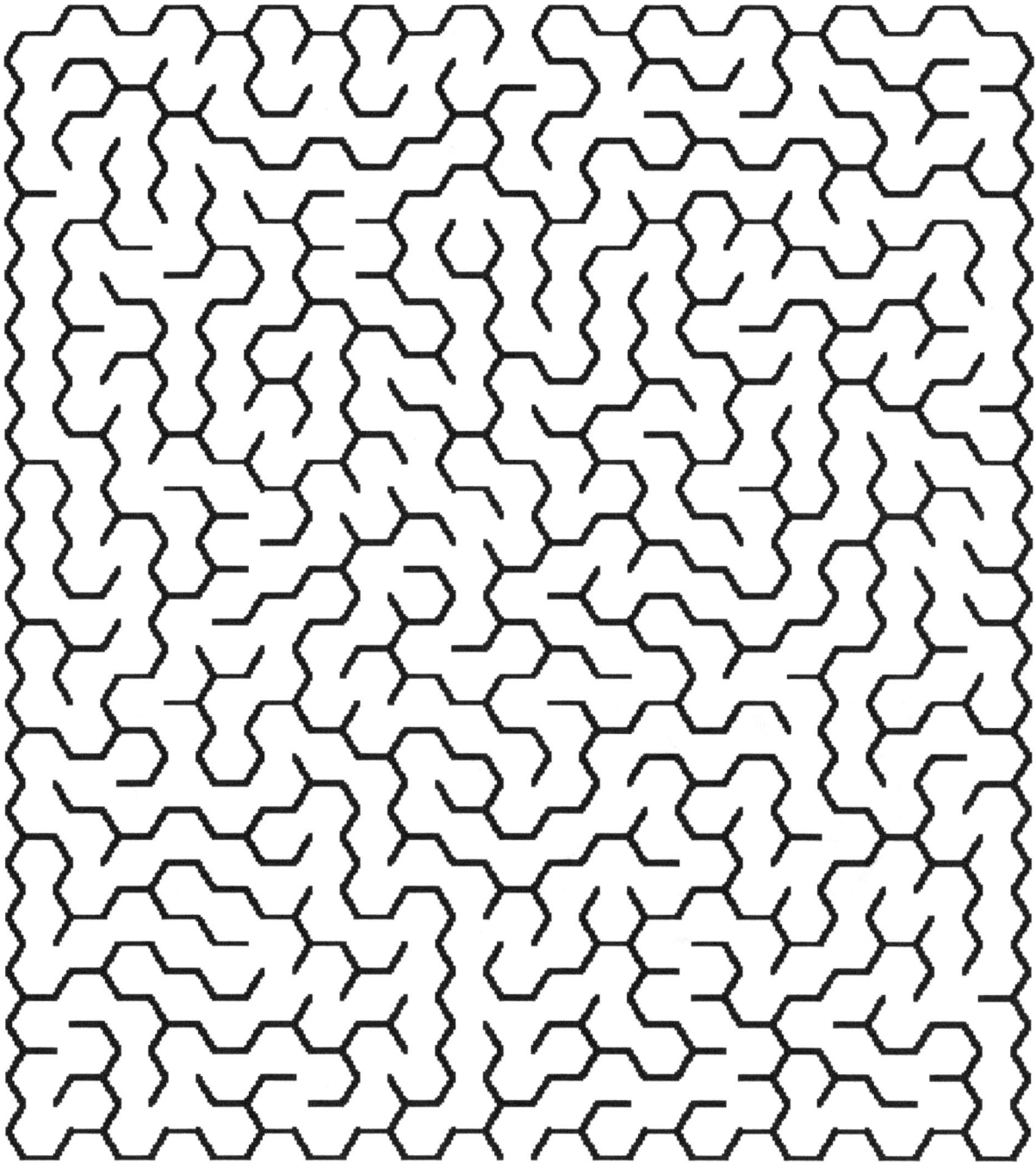

**Star**

Finish in the center.

**Star**

**Finish in the center.**

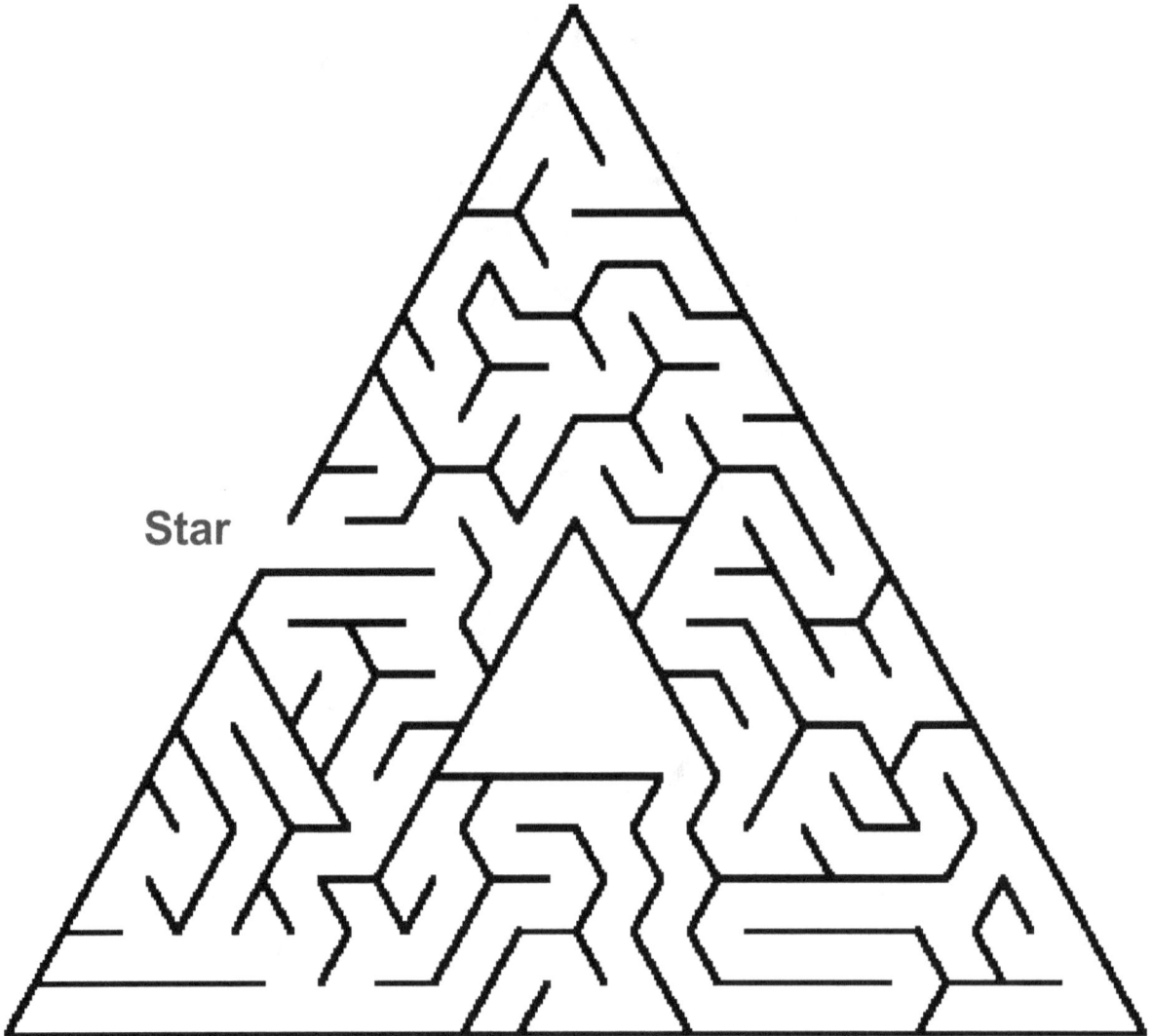

**Star**

Finish in the center.

**Start**

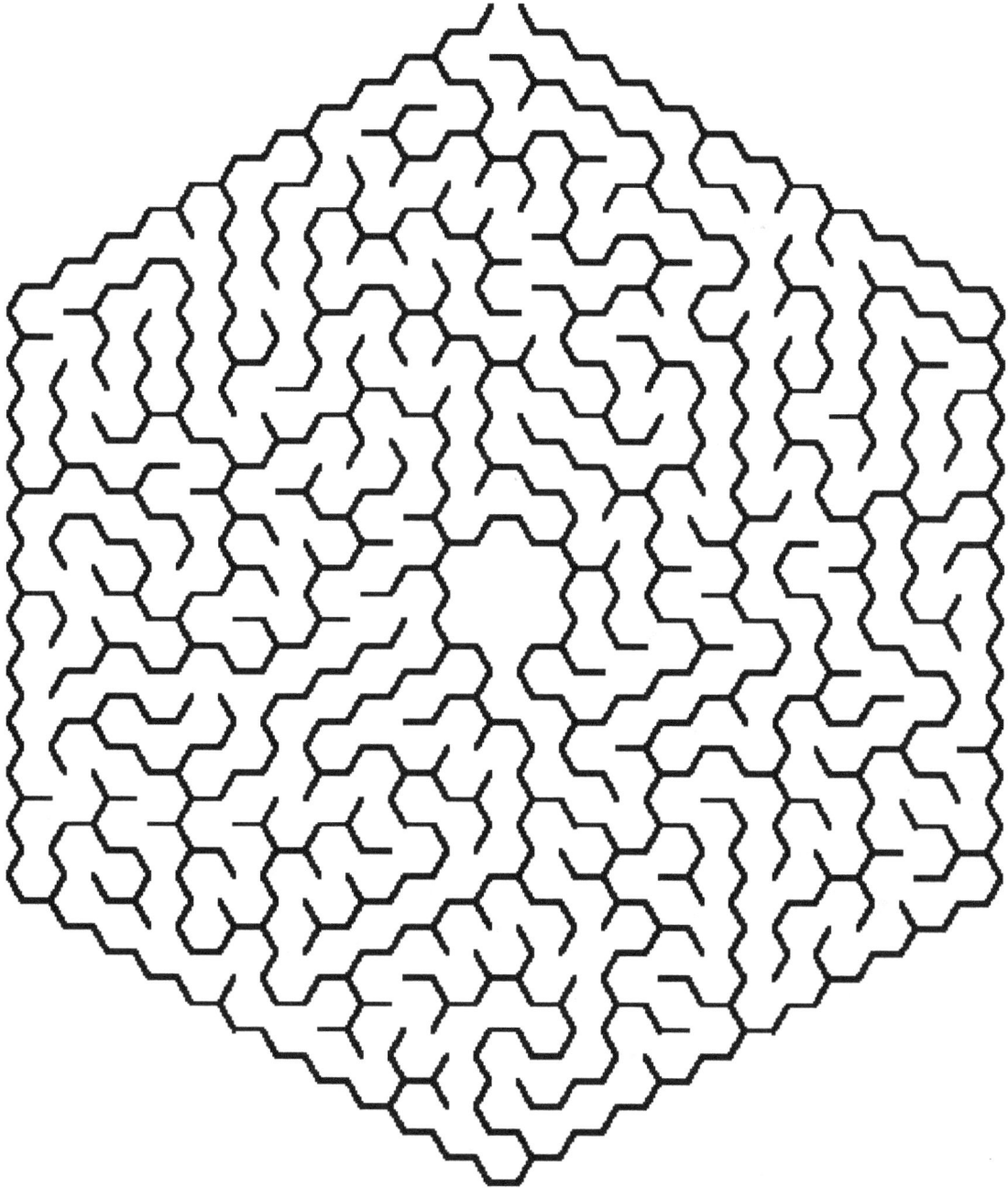

**Finish in the center.**

**Start**

**Finish in the center.**

**Start**

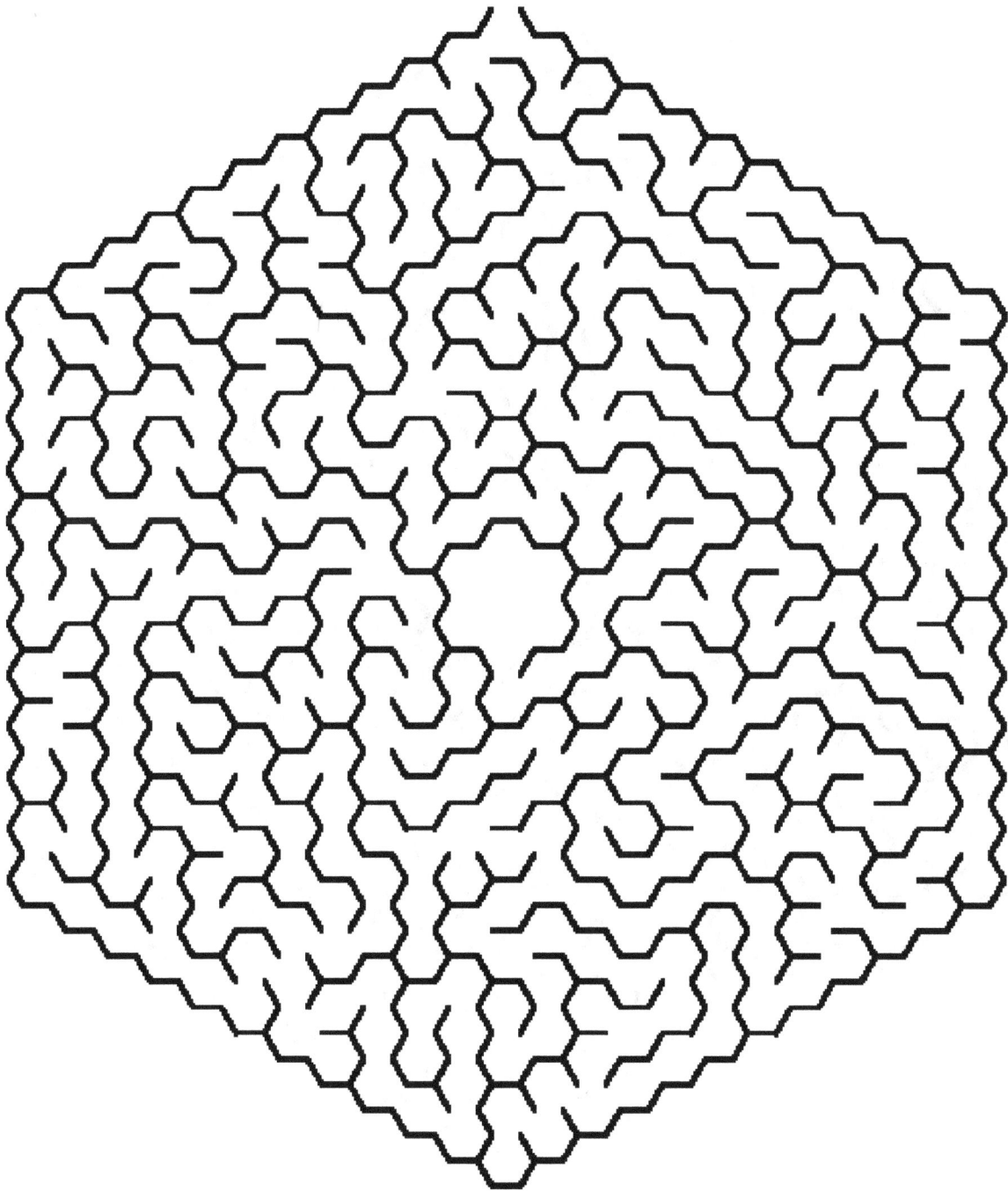

**Finish in the center.**

**Start**

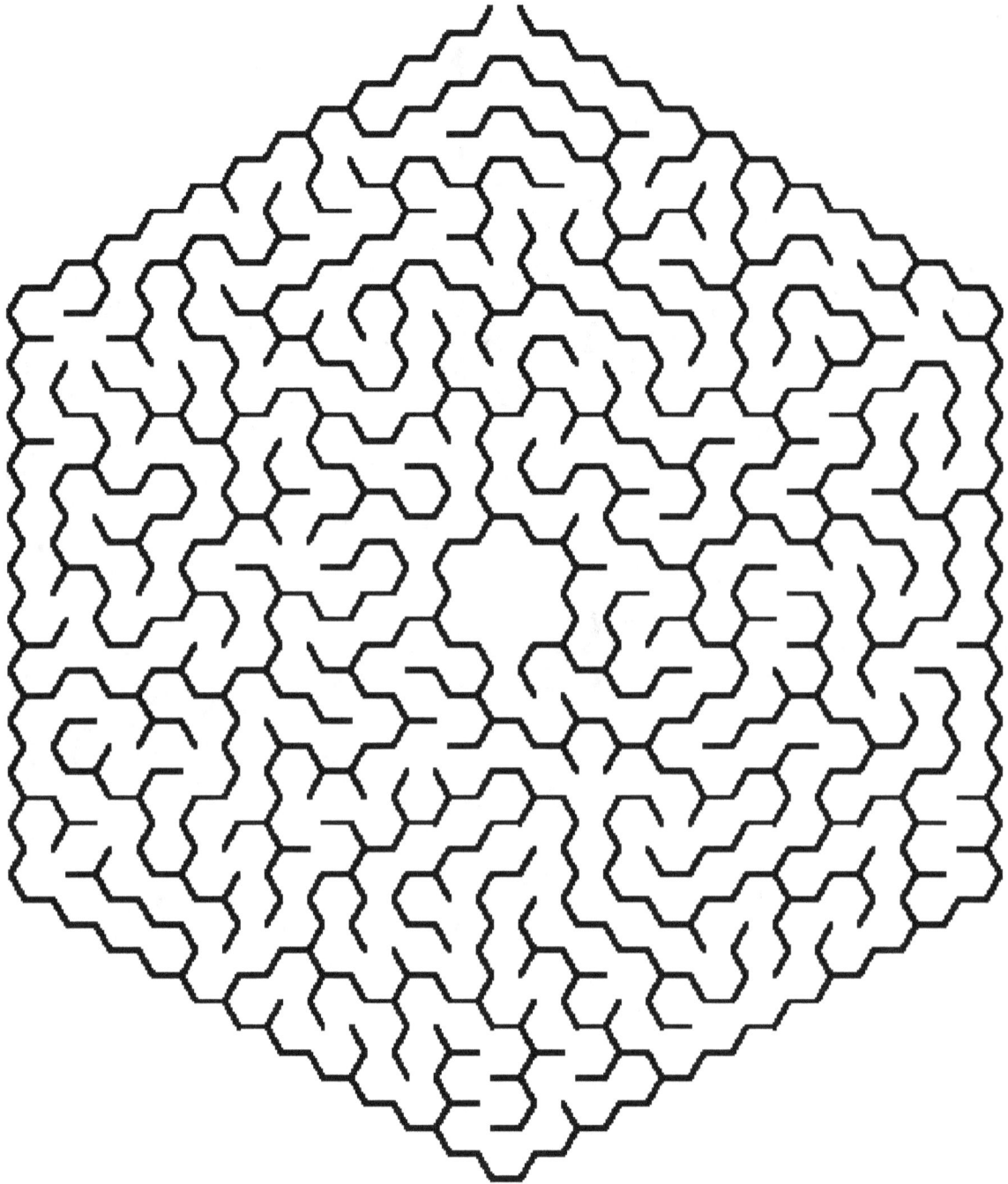

**Finish in the center.**

# Word Problems

Word problems are not only fun but also serve as excellent neurocognitive exercise because they engage multiple areas of the brain simultaneously. Solving them requires reading comprehension, logic, reasoning, and mathematical thinking—all of which challenge the brain to make connections, identify relevant information, and apply problem-solving strategies. This mental multitasking enhances executive functions, including working memory, attention control, and cognitive flexibility. Additionally, the real-world context of word problems adds an element of storytelling, making them more engaging and enjoyable, and further enhancing motivation and deeper learning.

Strengthening critical thinking skills is especially important for senior citizens, as it helps keep the mind sharp and supports independence in daily life. Whether it's deciding which medications to take and when, spotting potential scams, comparing prices at the store, or planning a balanced weekly schedule, critical thinking helps seniors make thoughtful, informed choices. It also improves memory, attention, and problem-solving skills that are key for managing health, finances, and social interactions. By practicing critical thinking, seniors can feel more confident, remain mentally engaged, and continue to participate in the world around them fully.

## Addition and Subtraction:

1. Sarah has 12 apples. She buys 8 more. How many apples does she have in total?

2. John had 25 marbles. He lost 7. How many marbles does he have now?

3. A farmer has 38 cows and sells 14. How many cows remain?

4. Lily had 45 candies and gave 19 to her friends. How many does she have left?

5. A store sold 23 hats in the morning and 17 in the afternoon. How many hats were sold in total?

6. A dog has 10 bones. A squirrel came along and stole 7 of them. How many bones does the dog have left?

## Multiplication:

7. A box contains 6 rows of chocolates, and each row has 8 chocolates. How many chocolates are there in total.

8. A school has 5 grades, and each grade has 22 students. How many students are in the school?

9. There are 9 chairs in each row and 7 rows in a hall. How many chairs are there in total?

10. A gardener plants 4 rows of trees, each row containing 15 trees. How many trees are planted?

11. A factory produces 12 cars per day. How many cars are made in 5 days?

12. A monkey eats 4 bananas per day. How many bananas will the monkey eat in one week?

13. A hat maker makes 2 hats per day. How many hats will the hat maker make in one year?

## Division:

14. 48 apples are divided equally among 8 children. How many apples does each child get?

15. A baker has 60 cupcakes and wants to pack them into boxes of 10. How many boxes will he need?

16. There are 35 pencils shared among 5 students. How many pencils does each student get?

17. A rope of 72 meters is cut into 9 equal pieces. What is the length of each piece?

18. A classroom of 30 students is divided into 6 equal groups. How many students are in each group?

19. A basketball game has two teams totaling 40 players. The teams are equally divided in half. How many are on each team?

## Mixed Operations:

20. Jenny bought 4 packs of pencils, each containing 10 pencils. She gave 12 away. How many pencils does she have left?

21. A farmer has 72 oranges and puts them into baskets of 8. How many baskets does he need?

22. A bookstore has 200 books. If 75 books are sold and 45 more arrive, how many books are in the store?

23. A restaurant prepares 9 tables with 6 chairs each. If 15 chairs are removed, how many chairs remain?

24. A worker earns $20 per hour. How much does he earn in 7 hours?

25. A football team has 9 players on the field until one gets injured and goes to the sidelines. Now how many are on the field?

## Time and Money:

26. If a movie starts at 3:30 PM and lasts for 2 hours and 15 minutes, what time does it end?

27. Emma bought 3 pens for $2 each and a notebook for $5. How much did she spend in total?

28. A train departs at 10:45 AM and reaches its destination at 2:30 PM. How long is the journey?

29. Tom has $50 and buys a toy for $27. How much money does he have left?

30. A worker starts his job at 9:15 AM and works for 6 hours. What time does he finish?

# Fractions:

31. Sarah ate 3/8 of a cake. How much of the cake is left?

32. A pizza is cut into 12 slices. If Tom eats 5 slices, what fraction of the pizza is left?

33. A classroom has 20 students, and 3/5 of them are girls. How many girls are there?

34. A baker uses 2/3 cup of sugar for a recipe. How much sugar is needed for 3 recipes?

35. A rope is 12 meters long. If 3/4 of it is used, how many meters remain?

## Percentages:

36. A shirt costs $40, and there is a 25% discount. What is the new price?

37. A student scores 80 out of 100 on a test. What percentage did they get?

38. A store increases prices by 10%. If a bag was $50, what is the new price?

39. A class has 30 students, and 40% are boys. How many boys are there?

40. A phone's battery is at 75%. If it originally had 2000 mAh, how much charge remains?

## Measurement and Area:

41. A rectangle has a length of 8 cm and a width of 5 cm. What is its area?

42. A car travels 60 miles in 2 hours. What is the speed per hour?

43. A field is 20 meters long and 15 meters wide. What is its area?

44. A cube has edges of 4 cm. What is its volume?

## Critical Thinking:

45. There are 3 baskets with a total of 36 apples. If one basket has twice as many as another, how are the apples divided?

46. If today is Wednesday, what day will it be in 15 days?

47. Two numbers add up to 50. One number is 14 more than the other. What are the numbers?

48. A train passes a 300-meter bridge in 15 seconds at a constant speed. What is the speed of the train?

# Math Problems

Math problems are not only fun but also an excellent way to keep the brain sharp and engaged. Solving math challenges requires logical thinking, pattern recognition, and concentration, all of which stimulate important areas of the brain. For many, the process of working through a problem and arriving at the correct answer brings a satisfying sense of achievement. Math puzzles, whether simple calculations or more complex word problems, provide a stimulating mental workout that can be both enjoyable and rewarding. They can be approached at any difficulty level, making them accessible and beneficial for seniors looking to keep their minds active.

For seniors, regularly practicing math can significantly improve cognitive functions used in everyday activities. Tasks like budgeting, measuring ingredients while cooking, calculating medication doses, or managing schedules all require basic math skills. Strengthening these abilities helps maintain independence and confidence in daily life. In addition, the problem-solving and critical thinking skills developed through math exercises support memory, attention span, and decision-making functions that tend to decline with age if not regularly exercised. By making math a fun and regular habit, seniors can support their brain health while staying sharp and capable in their daily routines.

**Addition:**

5 + 3 =

8 + 6 =

12 + 4 =

7 + 9 =

15 + 5 =

10 + 2 =

20 + 3 =

6 + 11 =

14 + 7 =

9 + 8 =

12 + 2 =

10 + 7 =

3 + 5 =

1 + 9 =

5 + 5 =

8 + 7 =

9 + 3 =

5 + 6 =

**Subtraction:**

10 - 4 =

15 - 7 =

20 - 5 =

8 - 3 =

12 - 6 =

18 - 9 =

25 - 10 =

30 - 15 =

14 - 8 =

9 - 2 =

7 - 3 =

6 - 1 =

10 - 7 =

4 - 2 =

5 - 1 =

7 - 5 =

8 - 3 =

4 - 1 =

**Multiplication:**

10 X 1 =

15 X 2 =

20 X 5 =

8 X 3 =

12 X  3 =

18 X  2 =

25 X 3 =

30 X 3 =

4 X 8 =

9 X  2 =

2 X 4 =

6 X 5 =

1 X 9 =

7 X 3 =

8 X 2 =

4 X 6 =

3 X 3 =

8 X 5 =

**Division:**

$10 \div 2 =$

$12 \div 3 =$

$15 \div 5 =$

$20 \div 4 =$

$18 \div 6 =$

$24 \div 8 =$

$30 \div 5 =$

$16 \div 4 =$

$9 \div 3 =$

$25 \div 5 =$

$8 \div 2 =$

$15 \div 5 =$

$9 \div 3 =$

$21 \div 7 =$

$36 \div 6 =$

$25 \div 5 =$

$80 \div 20 =$

$40 \div 5 =$

# Reminiscence Therapy & Conversation Cues

Reminiscence therapy is a person-centered approach that encourages individuals with Alzheimer's or dementia to recall and share meaningful memories from their past. By using photos, music, familiar scents, or objects from earlier life stages, this therapy can spark conversation, promote emotional connection, and enhance self-worth. Reminiscence therapy not only helps preserve a sense of identity but also provides comfort through the familiarity of long-term memories, which often remain accessible even as short-term memory fades.

Below are samples of questions you might ask during reminiscence therapy.

## Childhood & School

- What games did you play as a child?
- Do you remember your first school or a favorite teacher?
- What was your lunchbox like or your favorite school lunch?
- Did you have any pets when you were growing up?

## Family & Home Life

- Tell me about your parents or siblings—what were they like?
- What was your childhood home like? Can you describe it?
- Did your family have any special traditions or routines?

## Love & Relationships

- How did you meet your spouse or first love?
- Do you remember your wedding day or a special date?
- What advice would you give to someone getting married today?

## Work & Accomplishments

- What was your first job? What did you enjoy about it?

- Did you ever learn a trade or special skill?

- What are you most proud of in your life?

## Holidays & Traditions

- What was your favorite holiday, and how did you celebrate?

- Do you recall any family recipes or dishes you particularly enjoyed?

- Did your family do anything unique for birthdays or anniversaries?

## Music, Hobbies & Entertainment

- What kind of music did you listen to growing up?

- Did you go to dances, concerts, or movies? Which ones stood out?

- What hobbies did you enjoy—sewing, gardening, fishing?

## Everyday Life & Community

- What did a typical day look like when you were younger?

- Did you have a favorite community event?

- What stores, churches, or landmarks do you remember?

# Hand-Eye Coordination Exercises

Hand-eye coordination exercises are both fun and beneficial because they often involve engaging, interactive, and rewarding games or activities. Whether it's tossing a ball, playing a simple video game, drawing, or even doing crafts, these activities require the brain and body to work together, strengthening the connection between visual input and physical response. This kind of practice keeps the mind alert and the body responsive, offering a sense of play while improving essential motor and cognitive skills. For seniors, these activities provide a positive way to stay active, mentally stimulated, and entertained, which can also help improve mood and reduce stress.

The benefits of hand-eye coordination exercises extend well into daily life for seniors. Improved coordination helps with essential tasks such as pouring a cup of coffee, using utensils, buttoning a shirt, dialing a phone, or navigating uneven terrain while walking. As we age, these once-simple tasks can become more challenging, but regular coordination exercises help maintain and even restore those abilities. By keeping both the mind and body in sync, seniors can enhance their confidence, reduce the risk of falls or accidents, and maintain greater independence in their day-to-day activities.

## Exercise 1:

With both hands, start by tapping the tip of your thumb to the tip of your index finger, then tap the tip of your middle finger, then tap the tip of your ring finger, next pinky finger, and then go back the way you came.

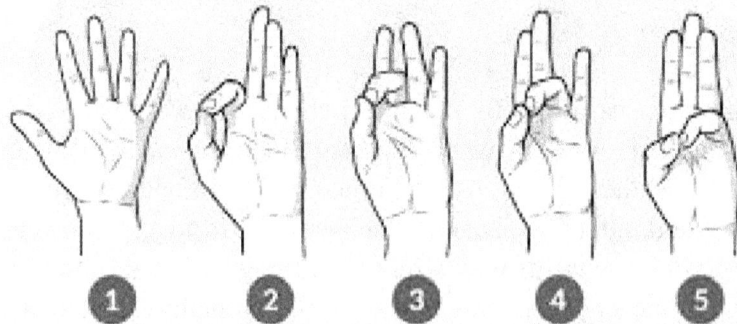

## Exercise 2:

Point your index finger from one hand and your pinky from the other toward each other and switch. The other fingers shouldn't move.

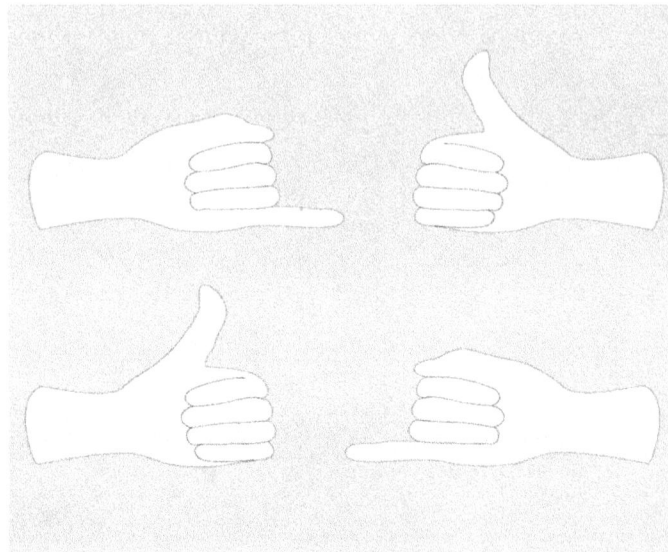

# Common Expressions!

Don't beat around the _____

It costs an arm and a _____

Once in a blue _____

By the skin of your _____

Don't cry over spilled _____

Don't count your chickens before they _____

Barking up the wrong _____

Don't beat around the _____

It's a blessing in _____

They are a dime a _____

Better late than _____

Let's call it a _____

Hit the _____

It's a piece of _____

A penny for your _____

Actions speak louder than _____

It only adds insult to _____

It won't cut the _____

You'll always get a second _____

Benefit of the _____

One bad apple won't spoil the _____

A picture is worth 1000 _____

You hit the nail on the _____

# Sensory Stimulation

Sensory stimulation can significantly enhance the quality of life for individuals with Alzheimer's and dementia. It taps into preserved senses and memories, promoting calm, joy, engagement, and connection—even when verbal communication becomes difficult. Below is a categorized list of effective sensory stimulation tools:

## Touch-Based Tools (Tactile)

- Fidget blankets or aprons – with zippers, buttons, fabrics, ribbons, beads

- Sensory balls – textured stress balls, squishy or spiky

- Soft fabric animals or dolls – for cuddling and comfort (lifelike therapy dolls or robotic pets)

- Weighted lap blankets or pads – provide calming pressure

- Hand massage kits – gentle oils and lotions to relax and soothe

- Kinetic sand or sensory bins – safe materials for digging, molding, and exploring

- Textured pillows or muffs – "Twiddle Muffs" with built-in tactile elements

## Scent-Based Tools (Olfactory)

- Aromatherapy diffusers – calming scents like lavender, peppermint, citrus, or rosemary

- Scented memory cards – to trigger reminiscence (e.g., pine, coffee, fresh-cut grass)

- Herb sachets – small cloth bags filled with cinnamon, cloves, or lavender

- Baking sessions – the scent of cookies or bread can be incredibly grounding and familiar

## Sound-Based Tools (Auditory)

- Personalized music playlists – favorite songs from their youth (helps trigger memory)

- Nature sounds – waves, rain, birdsong, wind chimes

- Chime therapy – soft wind or hand chimes to create a soothing atmosphere

- Talking photo albums – recordable voice messages with photos

- Interactive plush toys that respond to touch or sound

## Visual-Based Tools (Sight)

- Coloring books for adults, especially with large patterns and calming scenes

- Photo albums and memory boxes – with labeled family pictures or familiar places

- Digital photo frames – rotating photos with gentle transitions

- Aquarium or lava lamps – visually soothing and mesmerizing

- Brightly colored objects – to help with focus and mood stimulation

- Large-print or high-contrast signage helps with orientation and independence

## Taste-Based Tools (Gustatory)

- Flavor sampling – small tastes of favorite or nostalgic foods

- Lollipops or hard candy can bring comfort if swallowing is not impaired

- Cultural or holiday food tastings – to spark memories and connection

- Smooth-textured finger foods can encourage self-feeding and engagement

### Multi-Sensory Experiences

- Gardening therapy – smell of soil, touch of plants, visual beauty, outdoor sounds

- Baking or cooking together – taste, smell, touch, sight, and sound

- Spa day at home – soft lighting, calming music, massage, and pleasant scents

# Resources & Support

Many organizations exist solely to educate, inform, and support individuals and families navigating the challenges of Alzheimer's and dementia care. These organizations are often found in every state and community, offering localized assistance, including support groups, care consultations, respite resources, and educational materials. In addition to regional offerings, several major organizations operate on a national and even global scale, working to advance research, raise awareness, and improve the quality of life for those living with cognitive decline and their caregivers.

The internet has become an invaluable tool in connecting caregivers to these resources. Whether you're looking for a nearby memory care support group, downloadable legal documents, or the latest medical research, a wealth of trusted information is just a few clicks away. Online forums, helplines, webinars, and virtual communities can offer encouragement and guidance at any hour, helping caregivers feel less isolated and more empowered. To help you begin or deepen your journey, I've provided a few primary resources that can serve as trusted starting points.

## *Online Organizations*

### Alzheimer's Association alz.org

The Alzheimer's Association is the leading voluntary health organization dedicated to Alzheimer's care, support, and research. Founded in 1980, it provides education and resources for individuals living with Alzheimer's disease and other dementias, as well as for their families and caregivers. The organization also advocates for public policies and funds scientific research aimed at preventing, treating, and ultimately curing Alzheimer's.

### The Dementia Society of America dementiasociety.org

The Dementia Society of America is a nonprofit organization dedicated to raising awareness, providing education, and offering support to individuals and families affected by all forms of dementia. Through outreach programs, resources, and advocacy, the Society empowers communities to understand better and manage the challenges of cognitive decline.

### The National Institute of Health nih.gov

The National Institutes of Health (NIH) is the United States' premier medical research agency, dedicated to advancing scientific knowledge and improving health through biomedical and public health research. As part of the U.S. Department of Health and Human Services, the NIH supports and conducts groundbreaking research to prevent, diagnose, and treat diseases worldwide.

# *Support Groups*

### Alzheimer's Association Support Groups

Offers in-person and virtual support groups for caregivers and individuals living with dementia, facilitated by trained professionals. These groups provide a safe space for caregivers and individuals living with dementia to share experiences and receive guidance.

### Alzheimer's Foundation of America (AFA) Support Groups

Provides free support groups led by licensed social workers trained in dementia care. These groups are designed to help individuals and families cope with the challenges of Alzheimer's and related dementias.

### Dementia Mentors

Offers a unique mentorship program that connects individuals living with dementia with trained mentors who also have dementia, fostering peer support and shared experiences.

### Memory Cafés Directory at Dementia Friendly America dfamerica.org

Informal social gatherings for individuals with dementia and their caregivers provide a relaxed environment for social interaction and support.

### UCSF Memory and Aging Center Support Group

Specialized support for individuals diagnosed with young-onset Alzheimer's and their caregivers, offering education and emotional support.

# *Magazines & Periodicals*

### Alzheimer's TODAY Magazine

Published by the Alzheimer's Foundation of America, this magazine offers practical advice, personal stories, and wellness tips for caregivers and families.

### Preserving Your Memory® Magazine

An award-winning publication providing the latest information on Alzheimer's disease, caregiving strategies, and healthy living tips.

### Mirador Magazine

A dementia-friendly publication designed for individuals experiencing cognitive changes, offering engaging content and activities.

**Dementia Together Magazine**

Published by the Alzheimer's Society, this magazine features real-life stories, research updates, and practical advice for individuals affected by dementia.

## *Alzheimer's & Dementia Medical Journals*

**Alzheimer's & Dementia: The Journal of the Alzheimer's Association**

A leading peer-reviewed journal covering a wide range of dementia research, from basic science to clinical trials.

**Journal of Alzheimer's Disease**

Publishes research on various aspects of Alzheimer's disease, including biomarkers, therapeutic trials, and disease mechanisms.

**Journal of Dementia and Alzheimer's Disease**

An open-access journal focusing on all types of dementia, with particular interest in Alzheimer's disease.

**American Journal of Alzheimer's Disease & Other Dementias**

An open-access journal providing research on Alzheimer's disease and other dementias, including clinical studies and reviews.

# A Message in Closing From the Author

To all the caregivers, family members, and loved ones walking alongside someone with Alzheimer's or dementia, please know that your presence matters more than words can express. Even when memories fade and recognition slips away, the warmth of your voice, the kindness in your touch, and the rhythm of your care create a sense of safety and love that lingers far beyond the moment. You are doing sacred work. You are the memory-keepers, the advocates, the gentle anchors in an ever-shifting tide.

This journey is not easy, but you are not alone. Grace lives in the small things—in the repeated stories, the patient redirections, the quiet moments of connection. Even when it feels like you're unseen or unheard, your efforts are building a legacy of compassion. Keep showing up, keep loving with tenderness, and know that in your giving, you are lighting the way for them and the world.

I wish you light and love.

Sincerely,
Lisa A. Greenlee

# References

Alzheimer's Association. (2024). *2024 Alzheimer's disease facts and figures*. Alzheimer's & Dementia, 20(3), 325–473. https://doi.org/10.1002/alz.13705

(Use for general stats, stages, and diagnosis methods)

Selkoe, D. J., & Hardy, J. (2016). The amyloid hypothesis of Alzheimer's disease at 25 years. *EMBO Molecular Medicine*, 8(6), 595–608. https://doi.org/10.15252/emmm.201606210

(Cited for amyloid plaques)

Iqbal, K., Liu, F., Gong, C. X., & Grundke-Iqbal, I. (2010). Tau in Alzheimer's disease and related tauopathies. *Current Alzheimer Research*, 7(8), 656–664. https://doi.org/10.2174/156720510793611592

(Cited for neurofibrillary tangles)

Ott, A., Stolk, R. P., van Harskamp, F., Pols, H. A., Hofman, A., & Breteler, M. M. (1999). Diabetes mellitus and the risk of dementia: The Rotterdam Study. *Neurology*, 53(9), 1937–1937. https://doi.org/10.1212/WNL.53.9.1937

Cheng, G., Huang, C., Deng, H., & Wang, H. (2012). Diabetes as a risk factor for dementia and mild cognitive impairment: A meta-analysis of longitudinal studies. *Internal Medicine Journal*, 42(5), 484–491. https://doi.org/10.1111/j.1445-5994.2012.02758.x

Insulin Resistance and "Type III Diabetes" Hypothesis

de la Monte, S. M., & Wands, J. R. (2008). Alzheimer's disease is type 3 diabetes–evidence reviewed. *Journal of Diabetes Science and Technology*, 2(6), 1101–1113. https://doi.org/10.1177/193229680800200618

Farris, W., Mansourian, S., Chang, Y., Lindsley, L., Eckman, E. A., Frosch, M. P., ... & Selkoe, D. J. (2003). Insulin-degrading enzyme regulates the levels of insulin, amyloid β-protein, and the β-amyloid precursor protein intracellular domain in vivo. *Proceedings of the National Academy of Sciences*, 100(7), 4162–4167. https://doi.org/10.1073/pnas.0230450100

Griffin, R. J., Moloney, A., Kelliher, M., Johnston, J. A., Ravid, R., Dockery, P., ... & O'Neill, C. (2005). Activation of Akt/PKB, increased phosphorylation of Akt substrates and loss and altered distribution of Akt and PTEN are features of Alzheimer's disease pathology. *Journal of Neurochemistry*, 93(1), 105–117. https://doi.org/10.1111/j.1471-4159.2004.03081.x

Craft, S., Baker, L. D., Montine, T. J., Minoshima, S., Watson, G. S., Claxton, A., ... & Gerton, B. (2012). Intranasal insulin therapy for Alzheimer's disease and amnestic mild cognitive impairment: A pilot clinical trial. *Archives of Neurology*, 69(1), 29–38. https://doi.org/10.1001/archneurol.2011.233.

Leqembi and New Alzheimer's Treatments

Eisai Co., Ltd. & Biogen Inc. (2023). *Leqembi (lecanemab-irmb) Prescribing Information.* U.S. Food and Drug Administration. https://www.accessdata.fda.gov

Van Dyck, C. H., Swanson, C. J., Aisen, P., Bateman, R. J., Chen, C., Gee, M., ... & Budd Haeberlein, S. (2023). Lecanemab in early Alzheimer's disease. *New England Journal of Medicine*, 388(1), 9–21. https://doi.org/10.1056/NEJMoa2212948

(Phase 3 Clarity AD trial for

Leqembi) Lifestyle & Non-Drug

Interventions

Morris, M. C., Tangney, C. C., Wang, Y., Sacks, F. M., Bennett, D. A., & Aggarwal, N. T. (2015). The MIND diet is associated with reduced incidence of Alzheimer's disease. *Alzheimer's & Dementia*, 11(9), 1007–1014. https://doi.org/10.1016/j.jalz.2014.11.009

(For lifestyle interventions like DASH and Mediterranean diet)

Gitlin, L. N., Marx, K., Stanley, I. H., & Hodgson, N. A. (2015). Translating evidence-based dementia caregiving interventions into practice: State-of-the-science and next steps. *The Gerontologist*, 55(2), 210–226. https://doi.org/10.1093/geront/gnu123

(For quality of life and caregiver focus)

Albert, M. S., et al. (2011). *The diagnosis of mild cognitive impairment due to Alzheimer's disease: Recommendations from the National Institute on Aging-Alzheimer's Association workgroups.* Alzheimer's & Dementia, 7(3), 270–279.

Alzheimer's Association. (2024). *2024 Alzheimer's Disease Facts and Figures.* https://www.alz.org

Birks, J. (2006). *Cholinesterase inhibitors for Alzheimer's disease.* Cochrane Database of Systematic Reviews.

Iqbal, K., Liu, F., Gong, C. X., & Grundke-Iqbal, I. (2010). *Tau in Alzheimer's disease and related tauopathies.* Biochimica et Biophysica Acta (BBA) - Molecular Basis of Disease, 1792(7), 672–681.

Jack, C. R., et al. (2018). *NIA-AA Research Framework: Toward a biological definition of Alzheimer's disease.* Alzheimer's & Dementia, 14(4), 535–562.

McShane, R., et al. (2019). *Memantine for dementia.* Cochrane Database of Systematic Reviews.

Selkoe, D. J., & Hardy, J. (2016). *The amyloid hypothesis of Alzheimer's disease at 25 years.* EMBO Molecular Medicine, 8(6), 595–608.

Sperling, R. A., et al. (2011). *Toward defining the preclinical stages of Alzheimer's disease: Recommendations from the National Institute on Aging.* Alzheimer's & Dementia, 7(3), 280–292.

Woods, B., et al. (2012). *Cognitive stimulation to improve cognitive functioning in people with dementia.* Cochrane Database of Systematic Reviews.

World Health Organization. (2023). *Dementia.*
https://www.who.int/news-room/fact-
heets/detail/dementia

Ott, A., et al. (1999). Diabetes mellitus and the risk of dementia: The Rotterdam Study. *Neurology*, 53(9), 1937–1942.

Cheng, G., et al. (2012). Type 2 diabetes as a risk factor for dementia in the elderly: A meta-analysis of prospective cohort studies. *Diabetes Research and Clinical Practice*, 97(3), 401–407.

De la Monte, S.M., & Wands, J.R. (2008). Alzheimer's disease is type 3 diabetes–evidence reviewed. *Journal of Diabetes Science and Technology*, 2(6), 1101–1113.

Farris, W., et al. (2003). Insulin-degrading enzyme regulates the levels of insulin, amyloid beta-protein, and the beta-amyloid precursor protein intracellular domain in vivo. *Proceedings of the National Academy of Sciences*, 100(7), 4162–4167.

Griffin, R.J., et al. (2005). Effects of the Alzheimer's disease-linked apolipoprotein E4 allele on insulin signaling in the brain. *The Journal of Biological Chemistry*, 280(10), 3761–3767.

Craft, S., et al. (2012). Intranasal insulin therapy for Alzheimer disease and amnestic mild cognitive impairment: a pilot clinical trial. *Archives of Neurology*, 69(1), 29–38.

FDA Approval and Regulatory Status
U.S. Food and Drug Administration. (2023, July 6). FDA Converts Novel Alzheimer's Disease Treatment to Traditional Approval. Retrieved from Alzheimer's Association. (2023, July 6). Alzheimer's Association Welcomes U.S. FDA Traditional Approval of Leqembi.

Clinical Trial Data
Van Dyck, C. H., Swanson, C. J., Aisen, P., et al. (2022). Lecanemab in Early Alzheimer's Disease. New England Journal of Medicine, 388(1), 9–21. doi:10.1056/NEJMoa2212948.

Eisai Inc. (2025, May). Leqembi® (lecanemab-irmb) is the First Medicine that Slows Progression of Alzheimer's Disease.

Maintenance Dosing Approval
Biogen Inc. (2025, January 26). FDA Approves LEQEMBI® (lecanemab-irmb) IV Maintenance Dosing for the Treatment of Early Alzheimer's Disease.

Neurology Live. (2025, January 26). FDA Approves New IV Maintenance Dosing for Alzheimer Treatment Leqembi.

Side Effects and Safety Profile
Medical News Today. (2023, July 6). Leqembi Side Effects and How to Manage Them.
Mayo Clinic. (2025, April). Lecanemab-irmb (Intravenous Route).

Access and Implementation Challenges
Verywell Health. (2025, February 15). Why It's Hard for Patients to Get the Newest Alzheimer's Drugs.


Clare, L., & Woods, R. T. (2004). Cognitive training and cognitive rehabilitation for people with early-stage Alzheimer's disease: A review. *Neuropsychological Rehabilitation*, 14(4), 385–401. https://doi.org/10.1080/09602010443000074

Sitzer, D. I., Twamley, E. W., & Jeste, D. V. (2006). Cognitive training in Alzheimer's disease: A meta-analysis of the literature. *Acta Psychiatrica Scandinavica*, 114(2), 75–90. https://doi.org/10.1111/j.1600-0447.2006.00789.x

Bahar-Fuchs, A., Clare, L., & Woods, B. (2013). Cognitive training and cognitive rehabilitation for mild to moderate Alzheimer's disease and vascular dementia. *Cochrane Database of Systematic Reviews*, (6). https://doi.org/10.1002/14651858.CD003260.pub2

Willis, S. L., Tennstedt, S. L., Marsiske, M., et al. (2006). Long-term effects of cognitive training on everyday functional outcomes in older adults. *JAMA*, 296(23), 2805–2814. https://doi.org/10.1001/jama.296.23.2805

Reijnders, J., van Heugten, C., & van Boxtel, M. (2013). Cognitive interventions in healthy older adults and people with mild cognitive impairment: A systematic review. *Ageing Research Reviews*, 12(1), 263–275. https://doi.org/10.1016/j.arr.2012.07.003

Tardif, S., & Simard, M. (2011). Cognitive stimulation programs in healthy elderly: A review. *International Journal of Alzheimer's Disease*, 2011, 378934. https://doi.org/10.4061/2011/378934

Belleville, S., Gilbert, B., Fontaine, F., Gagnon, L., Ménard, E., & Gauthier, S. (2006). Improvement of episodic memory in persons with mild cognitive impairment and healthy older adults: Evidence from a cognitive intervention program. *Dementia and Geriatric Cognitive Disorders*, 22(5-6), 486–499. https://doi.org/10.1159/000096316

Gates, N. J., & Sachdev, P. S. (2014). Is cognitive training an effective treatment for preclinical and early Alzheimer's disease? *Journal of Alzheimer's Disease*, 42(Suppl 4), S551–S559. https://doi.org/10.3233/JAD-141302

Smith, G. E., Housen, P., Yaffe, K., et al. (2009). A cognitive training program based on principles of brain plasticity: Results from the Improvement in Memory with Plasticity-based Adaptive Cognitive.


Training (IMPACT) study. *Journal of the American Geriatrics Society*, 57(4), 594–603. https://doi.org/10.1111/j.1532-5415.2008.02167.x

Ball, K., Berch, D. B., Helmers, K. F., et al. (2002). Effects of cognitive training interventions with older adults: A randomized controlled trial. *JAMA*, 288(18), 2271–2281. https://doi.org/10.1001/jama.288.18.2271

Alzheimer's Association. (n.d.). Daily care plan. Retrieved July 16, 2025, from https://www.alz.org/help-support/caregiving/daily-care/daily-care-planAlzheimer's Association+2Alzheimer's Association+2Alzheimer's Association+2

Alzheimer's Association. (n.d.). Food & eating. Retrieved July 16, 2025, from https://www.alz.org/help-support/caregiving/daily-care/food-eatingAlzheimer's Association

Alzheimer's Association. (n.d.). Medication safety. Retrieved July 16, 2025, from https://www.alz.org/help-support/caregiving/safety/medication-safetyAlzheimer. Alzheimer's Association.

Alzheimer's Society. (n.d.). Taking medications with dementia. Retrieved July 16, 2025, from https://www.alzheimers.org.uk/about-dementia/treatments/dementia-medication/taking-dementia-medicati onsAlzheimer's Society

Alzheimer's Society. (n.d.). How does dementia affect washing and dressing? Retrieved July 16, 2025, from https://www.alzheimers.org.uk/get-support/daily-living/washing-dressingAlzheimer's Society

Alzheimer's Society. (n.d.). Therapy and approaches for supporting memory loss. Retrieved July 16, 2025, from https://www.alzheimers.org.uk/about-dementia/stages-and-symptoms/symptoms/approaches-therapy-mem ory-lossAlzheimer's Society+1Alzheimer's Society+1

Alzheimer's Society. (n.d.). Reducing and managing behaviour that challenges. Retrieved July 16, 2025, from https://www.alzheimers.org.uk/about-dementia/stages-and-symptoms/dementia-symptoms/managing-beha viour-changesThe Scottish Sun+3Alzheimer's Society+3Alzheimer's Society+3

Alzheimer's Society. (n.d.). Understanding and Supporting a Person with Dementia Retrieved July 16, 2025, from https://www.alzheimers.org.uk/get-support/help-dementia-care/understanding-supporting-person-dementi aAlzheimer's Society

Alzheimer's Society. (n.d.). Dementia and personal hygiene. Retrieved July 16, 2025, from https://www.dementiauk.org/information-and-support/health-advice/dementia-and-personal-hygiene/Dem entia UK

BrightFocus Foundation. (n.d.). Developing a dementia care plan. Retrieved July 16, 2025, from https://www.brightfocus.org/resource/developing-a-dementia-care-plan/BrightFocusFoundation

National Institute on Aging. (n.d.). Alzheimer's caregiving: Bathing, dressing, and grooming. Retrieved July 16, 2025, from https://www.nia.nih.gov/health/alzheimers-caregiving/alzheimers-caregiving-bathing-dressing-and-groom ingNational Institute on Aging

National Institute on Aging. (n.d.). Caring for older patients with cognitive impairment. Retrieved July 16, 2025, from https://www.nia.nih.gov/health/health-care-professionals-information/caring-older-patients-cognitive-imp airmentNational Institute on Aging

Practical Neurology. (n.d.). Behavioral approaches in dementia care. Retrieved July 16, 2025, from https://practicalneurology.com/diseases-diagnoses/alzheimer-disease-dementias/behavioral-approaches-in
-dementia-care/31800/Practical Neurology

ESPEN guideline on nutrition and hydration in dementia. (2024). Clinical Nutrition, S0261-5614(24)00146-8. Retrieved July 16, 2025, from https://www.clinicalnutritionjournal.com/article/S0261-5614%2824%2900146-8/fulltextClinical Nutrition Journal+1ScienceDirect+1

Reducing the risk of falls for people with dementia. (n.d.). Alzheimer's Society of Manitoba. Retrieved July 16, 2025, from https://www.alzheimer.mb.ca/wp-content/uploads/2013/09/2014-Dementia-Fall-Risk-Checklist-template. pdfAlzheimer. Alzheimer's Society of Manitoba

Dementia Care Plan: A Guide for Caregivers. (n.d.). National Council of Certified Dementia Practitioners. Retrieved July 16, 2025, from https://www.nccdp.org/dementia-care-plan-guide-for-caregivers/NCCDP

# Author Biography

**Author Lisa A. Greenlee** is a Geriatric Nurse Care Manager, Certified Dementia Practitioner, & Cognitive Health Program Consultant. She has dedicated her entire nursing career to improving the quality of life for older adults and their families.

Lisa is a trusted member of the healthcare community in central Ohio, fostering inclusivity through client-centered, family-focused engagement. She has established strong working relationships with geriatricians and specialty care physicians, ensuring collaborative and comprehensive care for her clients.

Lisa has also trusted relationships with elder law attorneys, trust attorneys, and wealth management professionals, who consistently rely on her expertise to support their aging clients. Recognized for her integrity and compassionate approach, she is often called upon to provide navigation, advocacy, and tailored care services that align with each client's legal, financial, and healthcare needs while preserving their dignity, autonomy, and quality of life.

As a Nurse Care Manager and Certified Dementia Practitioner, Lisa focuses on *person-centered care planning* to meet social-emotional needs in order to preserve quality of life and dignity of her clients. Her specialized care plan approach also monitors the progression of the disease process to adjust interventions accordingly.

In her role as a Cognitive Health Program Consultant, she teaches family and caregiver support, educates families on the stages of dementia and care techniques, and advises on how to provide emotional support and access resources to reduce caregiver burnout.

Lisa is the founder of **Benchmark Nursing Solutions, LLC**, a concierge nurse care management company, and the creator of **SPARK© Neurocognitive Model of Care**, a program designed to support and empower caregivers with care plans that help ensure safety while making quality of life central. Other published works include: **Beacon of Light – Guided Journal**, *52 Weeks of Intention: A Reflective Journey Through Affirmation, Stillness, and Gratitude,* and **Firefly Faith – Little Lights That Lead Us**, *A Pocket Devotional for the Weary & Faithful.*

In her private life, Lisa is a published author and painter, actively engaged in the arts. She resides in Circleville, Ohio, and is especially devoted to her family and friends.

Lisa believes living a life in service of others is imperative for the soul because it connects us to something greater than ourselves. Acts of compassion and kindness awaken empathy, deepen our sense of purpose, and nurture inner peace. Service dissolves isolation and invites meaning, reminding us that the soul thrives not in self-interest but in selfless giving.

*"In lifting others, we rise."*

*www.lisagreenlee.com*

*www.benchmarknursingsolutions.com*

www.ingramcontent.com/pod-product-compliance
Lightning Source LLC
Chambersburg PA
CBHW081417270326
41931CB00015B/3302

# An Introduction of Me

My name: _____

My address: _____

_____

My phone number: _____

**My Class information:**

Homeroom Teacher: _____

Room: _____

School year: _____

My student ID: _____

**Emergency Contact information:**

Name:

_____

Relationship to Student: _____

Telephone: _____

Email: _____

Name:

_____

Relationship to Student: _____

Telephone: _____

Email: _____

**Known Allergies:** _____

_____

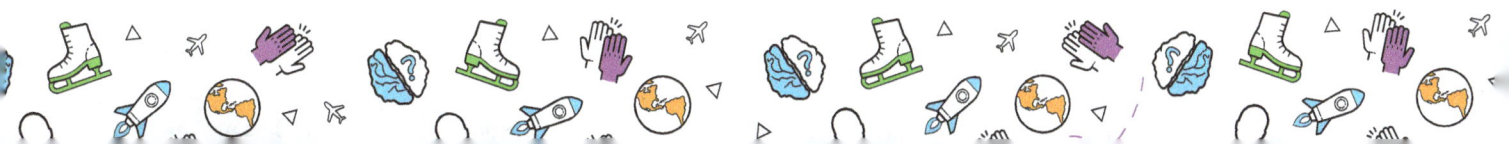

# An Introduction of Me

**My favorites:**

Color: _____

Book: _____

Song: _____

Movie: _____

Food: _____

Hobby: _____

Sport: _____

I'm unique because _____

_____

_____

_____

_____

_____

_____

Below, write a letter to yourself about how you're feeling at the start of this new year and what you are looking forward to throughout the year. (You can then revisit this letter at the end of the year.)

_____

_____

_____

_____

_____

_____

_____

_____

_____

_____

# Using This Planner 1

Welcome to your planner!

This planner is a place for you to write and organize your homework, plan out your extracurricular activities, and manage your time well. It is also a place for you to learn and practice your social emotional learning (SEL) skills. Throughout this planner you will learn how to:

## LEARN SELF-AWARENESS

Accurately recognize your emotions, thoughts, and values; and develop a growth mindset.

## LEARN SELF-MANAGEMENT

Regulate your emotions, thoughts, and behaviors, manage your stress, and set goals for yourself.

## LEARN RELATIONSHIP-SKILLS

Create and maintain friendship, communicate well with others, and resist negative peer pressure.

## LEARN RESPONSIBLE DECISION-MAKING

Identify and solve problems, reflect, and consider the well-being of yourself and others.

## LEARN SOCIAL-AWARENESS

Respect all people, take others' perspectives into account, and empathize with others.

Make connections between each skill and books or other texts you have read at school or at home.

Explore each of the skills above in theme pages with activities to explore each skill (competency) at the end of the theme. Review each skill theme more fully.

In this planner you will also:

A check-list to determine what you still need to work on, and what you feel confident about in regards to SEL.

Trackers to help you remember the activities and service learning you complete this year.

Stories of students like you who solved their problems using their SEL skills.

Self-Care toolkits to give you ideas on how to take care of your own well-being.

Calming exercises to help lessen your stress.

How to use SEL in your daily life.

At the end of this planner, you will find pages to help you continue learning your SEL skills.

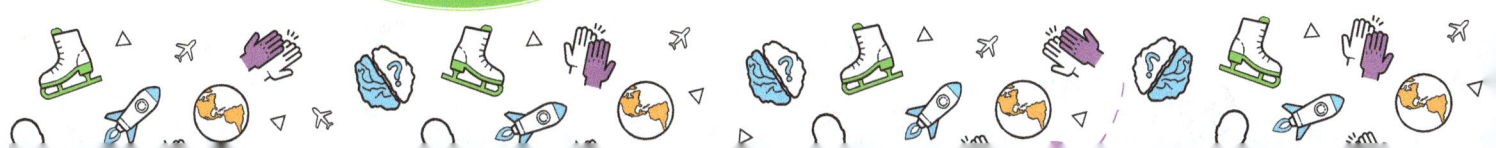

# Using This Planner II

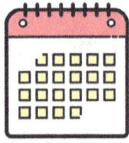

**The Activities:**

This planner provides you with opportunities to practice the skills you are learning using real-life examples and giving you the opportunity to reflect on your learning. Activities will vary between whole group lessons, small groups, individual activities, activities to do at home, or activities to do at school.

## WEEKS 1-10
### IDENTITY & MINDSET

## WEEKS 11-20
### COURAGE & KINDNESS

## WEEKS 21-30
### A PLACE TO BELONG

## WEEKS 31-40
### A HEALTHY WELL-BEING

**Resume Builder:**

A chart in the back of this planner where you can record all the activities, sports, clubs, and volunteer programs you are involved in this year to help you build your resume for college applications, scholarships, and other special programs.

**Creative Expression:**

Pages for you to focus and be mindful in the present moment.

Use them when you need to focus and listen while keeping your hands busy, or you want to destress and have a quiet moment.

**Review weeks:**

The planner gives you the time and space to think about your learning throughout the past 9 weeks, and give you a place to practice building on the skills you are learning.

**Service Learning:**

A chart where you can track all your service learning throughout the year. This is helpful if your school requires you to complete a certain number of service hours each year as well as provides documentation of your service for future scholarships.

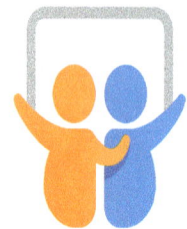

# FOR PARENTS AND CARERS:

YOU CAN SHARE WHAT YOU ARE LEARNING WITH YOUR PARENTS OR CARER AT HOME TOO. THE ADULTS IN YOUR LIFE WANT YOU TO FEEL GOOD ABOUT YOURSELF, LEARN MORE ABOUT HOW YOUR BRAIN AND HEART RESPOND TO THINGS, AND HAVE FRIENDS WHO YOU CAN RELY ON!

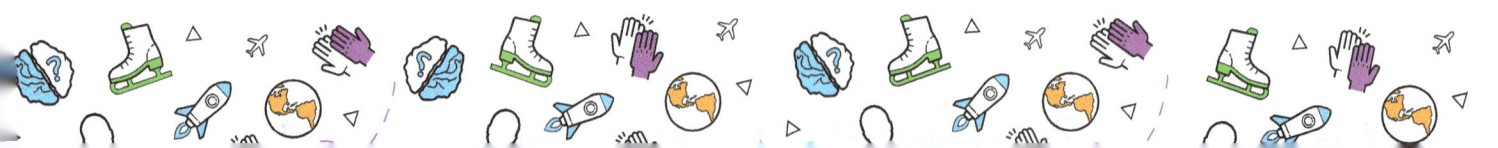

# Common Content

## Term 1

| Period / Hour | Subject | Room # | Teacher |
|---|---|---|---|
| | | | |
| | | | |
| | | | |
| | | | |
| | | | |
| | | | |
| | | | |
| | | | |

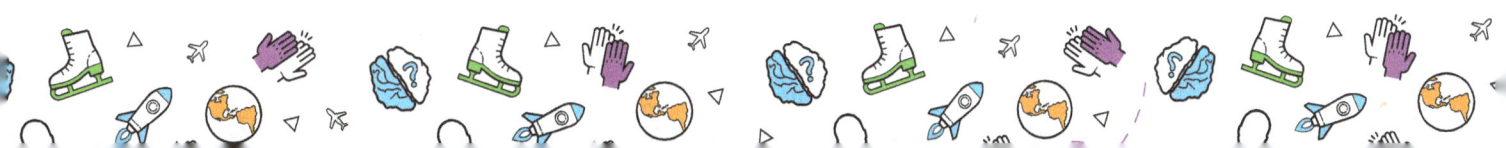

## Term 2

| Period / Hour | Subject | Room # | Teacher |
|---|---|---|---|
| | | | |
| | | | |
| | | | |
| | | | |
| | | | |
| | | | |
| | | | |
| | | | |

## Term 3

| Period / Hour | Subject | Room # | Teacher |
|---|---|---|---|
| | | | |
| | | | |
| | | | |
| | | | |
| | | | |
| | | | |
| | | | |
| | | | |

# Notes

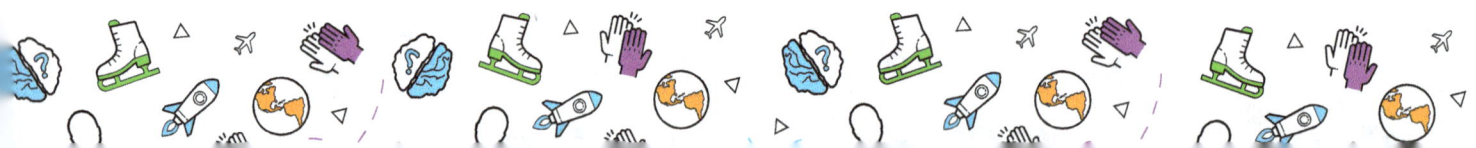

# Notes

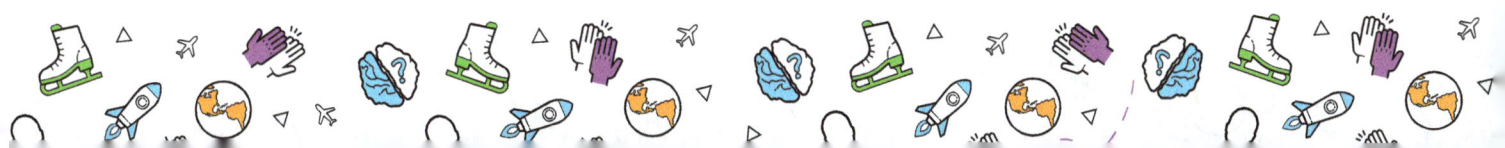

# Goals for 7th Grade

**#Goals** The beginning of a new school year can be a fresh new start, just like putting up a new calendar in January. You may have gone shopping for new supplies, shoes, or clothes and you may be sitting at your new desk with new pencils and pens, folders or notebooks. As a 7th grader, the start of school may not be such a big deal. You may be someone who is not excited about starting school. Maybe you have had a bad experience in the past. This is the perfect chance to put the past behind you and start fresh.

The new school year can be overwhelming. One way people can face new things is by setting goals for themselves. "I don't focus on what I'm up against. I focus on my goals, and I try to ignore the rest," said Venus Williams, star tennis player. Goals do not always have to be about being a great athlete or making the best grades. When I was in middle school, my goal was to be in the symphonic band class. Your goals may be more significant than that.

Goals require action, work, focus, and dedication to achieve your dreams. Let's say you want to be an actor, lawyer, or a basketball player. You don't just show up one day, and you're automatically a success, you have to take steps to get there. Think of all the famous people, successful people, and people who have jobs or careers you might like to have one day. Once upon a time, they too were in middle school, sitting at a desk with new pens and paper just like you. How did they become successful? They had a dream, and they made their dream real by making goals for themselves. "A goal is a dream with a deadline." – Napoleon Hill

**Activity:** Think about what you would love to do; dream for a minute. These dreams can be for this school year, about activities you want to do like sports or band, about your grades or your attendance; they can even be about things outside of school. Take step #1 to making these dreams into goals by writing them down in the space below:

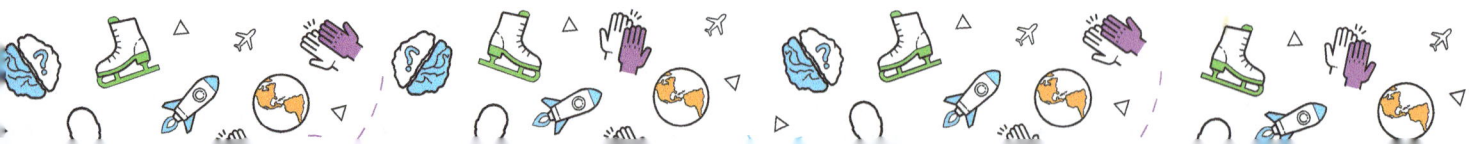

# Goals for 7th Grade

**Goal #1:** _____

_____

_____

_____

_____

_____

_____

_____

Date you will accomplish this goal: _____

Steps you will take to reach this goal:

1) _____

_____

2) _____

_____

3) _____

_____

How will you know you've accomplished this goal? _____

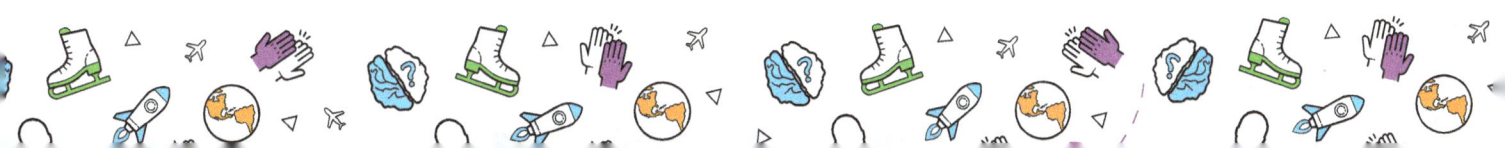

_____

_____

_____

_____

_____

_____

# Goals for 7th Grade

**Goal #2:** _____

_____

_____

_____

_____

_____

_____

_____

Date you will accomplish this goal: _____

Steps you will take to reach this goal:

1) _____

_____

2) _____

_____

3) _____

_____

How will you know you've accomplished this goal? _____

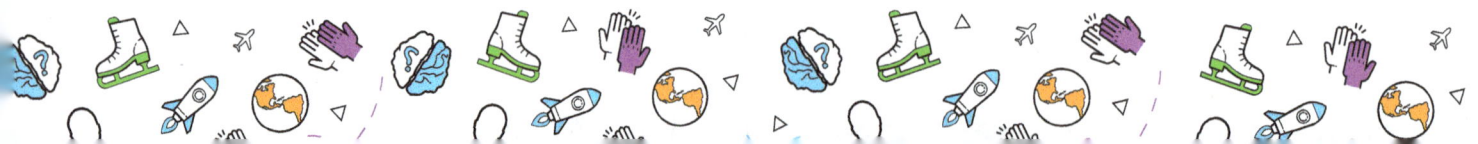

_____

_____

_____

_____

_____

_____

# Goals for 7th Grade

**Goal #3:** _____

_____

_____

_____

_____

_____

_____

Date you will accomplish this goal: _____

Steps you will take to reach this goal:

1) _____

_____

2) _____

_____

3) _____

_____

How will you know you've accomplished this goal? _____

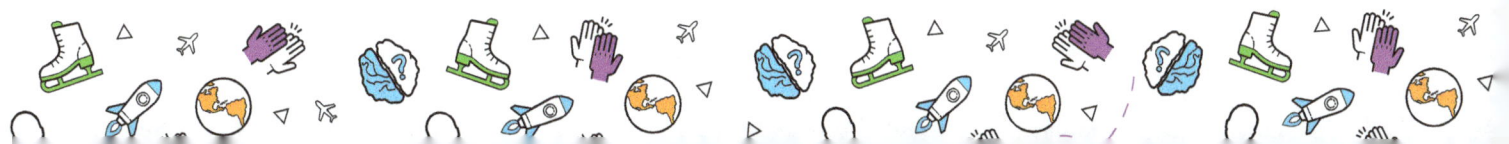

_____

_____

_____

_____

_____

_____

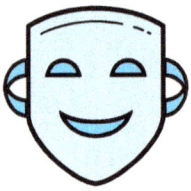

# Identity and Mindset

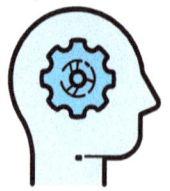

The next 10 weeks will focus on identity and mindset, with an emphasis on the social-emotional competency of self-awareness.

**Throughout this theme, you will be focusing on:**

1) Starting middle school with confidence and ease (Self-confidence)
2) Ways you learn best (Recognizing strengths & Accurate self-perception)
3) How your identity can change based on who you are with (Accurate self-perception)
4) Identifying and regulating various emotions (Identifying emotions)
5) Understanding what is in your control (Accurate self-perception & Self-efficacy)
6) Self-Talk and growth mindset (Self-confidence, Recognizing strengths, & Self-efficacy)

To introduce you to the themes of identity and mindset, we have given you some suggestions for something to read, listen to, and taste. Spend some time over the next ten weeks exploring this theme.

**Read:** From your school or community library, check out *Inside Out* and *Back Again* by Thanhha Lai. This book is about a young immigrant from Vietnam who comes to the USA. Journey with Ha, the main character, as she discovers her new identity in her new life. This novel is a great one for thinking about identity and mindset. Enjoy!

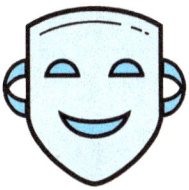

# Identity and Mindset

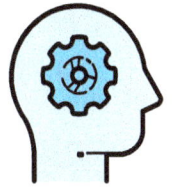

**Listen to:** With your carer's permission, go online to listen to "Lovely Day" by Bill Withers. This song is great to get you in a positive mindset and remind you that every day can be a lovely day with the right mindset.

When you wake up in the morning, what can remind you that it can be a lovely day? _____

_____

_____

What is your favorite line or part of this song? _____

_____

_____

How does this song make you feel? _____

_____

_____

**Taste:** Think about your favorite food. The theme these ten weeks is about learning about ourselves and how we have the ability to change our mindset and regulate our emotions: we get to control ourselves. Find time over the next few weeks to eat your favorite food.

My favorite food is _____

When I eat it, I feel _____

_____

This food feeds into my identity because _____

_____

# Welcome Back to Middle School! Who are you?

Identity is the distinguishing personality of an individual; identity is more than what we look like or who our family is. As a 7th grader who has overcome the beginning of middle school, who knows the ropes, your identity continues to be important. You may often look to your friends, social media, and celebrities to find cues as to what you like, what you think or feel about a variety of topics, and how to dress. Talking about and deciding who you are is not always easy. When we look to others to tell us how to be, our identity can change depending on the trends and what others want. Our best bet is to spend time making our own choices, working through different reflective questions, making responsible choices will help shape who we are over time. That way, who we are is consistent, and others will recognize us by our character and personality.

Think about some questions and reflect on your answers. Be true to yourself in how you answer.

- Who are some people who are important to you?
- What activities do you enjoy?
- What do you hope to accomplish this year? Next year? In your future?
- Describe your personality.
- What do you want in a friend?
- What books do you like? What movies? Music?
- What groups are you part of?
- What skills and talents do you have or are working on?

Remember you are always creating and developing your identity. As you grow and go through different stages, parts of your identity will grow and change with you, such as relationships, graduations, or jobs. Keep this in mind, and notice what values and ethics you demonstrate, and how you work through difficulties.

**Activity:** When you made your goals for the year, you were working on who you wanted to be at the end of the year! If you had an ingredients label that describes who you are, what would it say you are made of? Make a label for yourself that tells what you are made of. Here's an example of how you might want to organize your ingredients label:

**IDENTITY FACTS**
Personal Size - feet, inches
Years
Grade

-----------------------

Qualities
Hobbies
Relationships
Goals
Interests

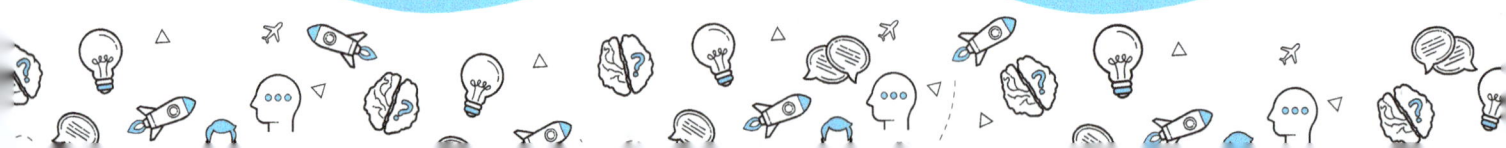

# Homework Log

Week beginning: ____ / ____ / ____

**My goal this week:** _____

_____

| | |
|---|---|
| **Monday** ___ / ___ | _____<br>_____<br>_____<br>_____ |
| **Tuesday** ___ / ___ | _____<br>_____<br>_____<br>_____ |
| **Wednesday** ___ / ___ | _____<br>_____<br>_____<br>_____ |
| **Thursday** ___ / ___ | _____<br>_____<br>_____<br>_____ |
| **Friday** ___ / ___ | _____<br>_____<br>_____<br>_____ |
| **Home/School Communication** | |

# Who Are You?

**Reminder:** Last week, you completed an activity that listed all the things that went into your personal identity. Did you have "Student" on your list? What percentage did you put of yourself as a student? It may have been a large percent. In fact, students spend a good portion of their time at school, doing homework, being involved in school activities, and participating in school sports, music, theater, or other extracurricular activities.

If you ask several students from any school, how they felt about school, you will get answers that fall along a line from "It's a way to get to where I want to go in life," "it's a job, something students have to do," to students who are disinterested and who are not motivated. Think about the beginning of this year when you started working on your goals for the year.

Research suggestions that students who view school as a way to help them meet their future goals, do the best in school and have a better experience than students who view school as a job or aren't interested in school. Where would you fall if you were part of this research study?

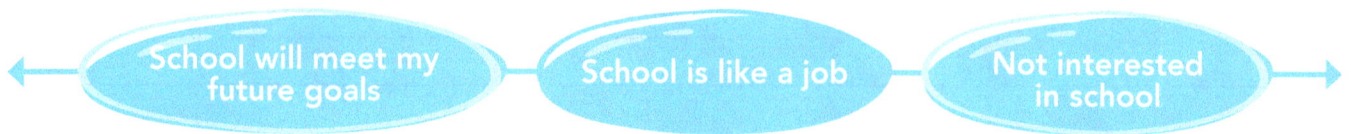

← —— ( School will meet my future goals ) —— ( School is like a job ) —— ( Not interested in school ) —— →

**Activity:** Remember, our identity evolves and changes as we do. If you find yourself on a spot on the line above that you are not comfortable with or wish you had a different identity as a learner, you can! Part of creating your identity as a learner is having the right frame of mind, encouraging yourself, getting help when you need it, and not giving up when things don't go well, or things are difficult. Reflect on where you are as a learner.

As a learner, I am _____

_____

_____

_____

Now go back to your goals to see if you need to make any changes or additions.

# Homework Log

Week beginning: ____ / ____ / ____

My goal this week: _____

_____

| | |
|---|---|
| **Monday** <br> ___ / ___ | _____ <br> _____ <br> _____ <br> _____ |
| **Tuesday** <br> ___ / ___ | _____ <br> _____ <br> _____ |
| **Wednesday** <br> ___ / ___ | _____ <br> _____ <br> _____ <br> _____ |
| **Thursday** <br> ___ / ___ | _____ <br> _____ <br> _____ |
| **Friday** <br> ___ / ___ | _____ <br> _____ <br> _____ <br> _____ |
| **Home/School Communication** | |

# The Identity Code

We have spent our time, so far, reflecting on our identity and about our identity as a learner. This week we are going to think about something called 'code-switching.' Think about your identity when you are with your friends versus your parents versus your teachers versus your grandparents.

How you are with your friends, or when you are by yourself, is likely very different than if you were in these other situations. You are still you, but what your reactions to social situations and your expectations in those environments change. You code-switch with different groups in order to project a particular identity. The change is usually based on the age of people you are with and location. We typically make the switch using social cues without even realizing it.

**Activity:** What changes, or code-switching, do you make in these situations?

| SITUATION: | WHAT MIGHT I NEED TO SWITCH UP? |
|---|---|
| Getting pizza with your teammates after practice. | |
| Shopping with friends. | |
| Volunteering at a nursing home. | |
| Meeting your favorite musician. | |
| Being told your curfew by your parents. | |
| Meeting with your school counselor. | |
| Talking with your teacher after class. | |
| Working with a group in class. | |

**Reminder:** Your identity is not what changes in code-switching situations. If you are a naturally shy person, you would still be a shy person no matter where you are or what is going on.

**Practice:** Learn the names of teachers, custodians, secretaries and greet them by their name, ask how they are, and smile. It will make their day, build a positive relationship with others, and will help practice code-switching.

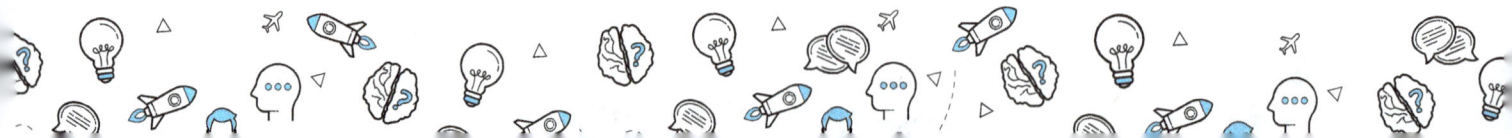

# Homework Log

Week beginning: ___ / ___ / ___

My goal this week: _____

_____

| | |
|---|---|
| **Monday**<br>___ / ___ | _____<br>_____<br>_____<br>_____ |
| **Tuesday**<br>___ / ___ | _____<br>_____<br>_____ |
| **Wednesday**<br>___ / ___ | _____<br>_____<br>_____<br>_____ |
| **Thursday**<br>___ / ___ | _____<br>_____<br>_____ |
| **Friday**<br>___ / ___ | _____<br>_____<br>_____<br>_____ |
| **Home/School Communication** | |

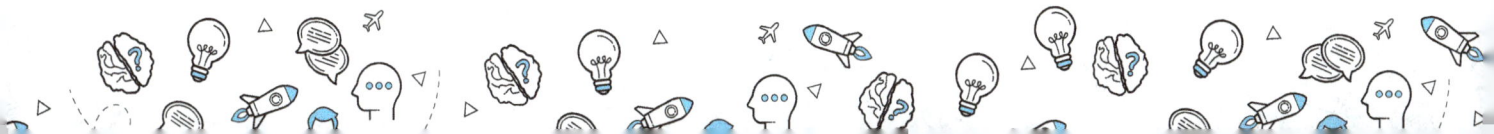

# More Than an Emoji

By the time students are in middle school, they have a good understanding of primary emotions like love, anger, fear, sadness, and joy. As a middle school student, you define your primary emotions often by 'liking/disliking" statements or photos, clicking a 🩵, or sharing a face to share how we feel 🙂. Other than expressing a basic like or dislike of something, are we truly communicating our emotions to others in a way that they understand, and in a way where we are sure others hear us? When we try to understand emotions in others, we can best do this by looking at the person, their face, their body language, and hearing their voice. The same is true when we want to understand our emotions better.

As we get older, our emotions change quickly, and it can be very confusing! In the 7th grade, we have moved past basic emotions and are recognizing new emotions that are more complex. Complex emotions are different from basic emotions because they are not always recognizable. They also require us to stop and think about our feelings and reflect on what is happening. For example, we may say something embarrassing, and your cheeks get red, and you look down, and you may want to disappear. Part of that emotion is fear. These complexities make it difficult to express ourselves and to understand the emotions of others.

**Activity:** With a partner, think about these more complex emotions, and identify *situations* when you experienced them. Talk with your partner about how your *body language*, *facial expression*, and *voice* sounds in each situation with each emotion.

**Confused (unknown + anxiety)**

**Frustrated**
**(annoyed + lack of confidence)**

**Overwhelmed (powerless + defeated)**

**Depressed (sad + helpless)**

**Jealous (mad + angry)**

**Disappointed (sad + loss)**

**Stress (worry + anxiety)**

**Guilty (sad+shame)**

**Annoyed (mad + irritated)**

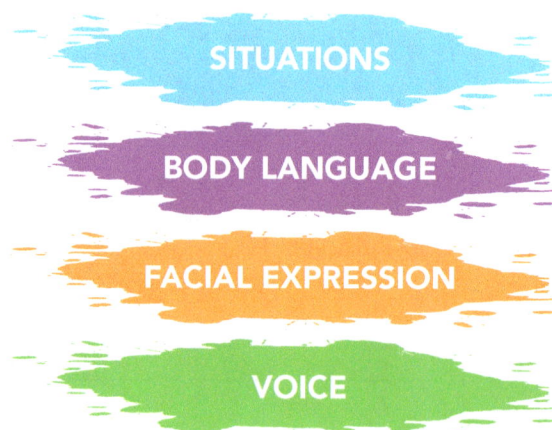

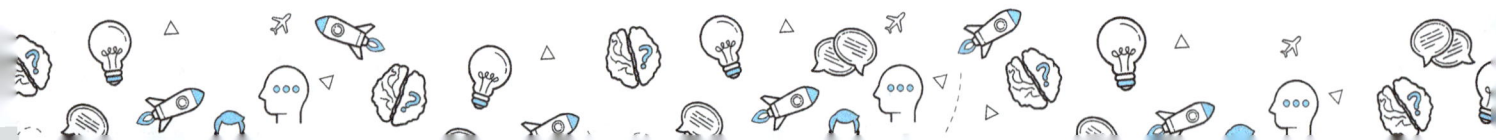

SITUATIONS

BODY LANGUAGE

FACIAL EXPRESSION

VOICE

# Homework Log

Week beginning: ____ / ____ / ____

My goal this week: _____

_____

| | |
|---|---|
| **Monday** <br> ___ / ___ | |
| **Tuesday** <br> ___ / ___ | |
| **Wednesday** <br> ___ / ___ | |
| **Thursday** <br> ___ / ___ | |
| **Friday** <br> ___ / ___ | |
| **Home/School Communication** | |

# I'm in Control

The key is to stay in control and regulate your emotions. Think of a dial turning the heat on a stove up or down. Our emotional responses tend to turn the dial up quickly. Our job is to be aware of this, be mindful, and turn the dial down on our before they get turned up all the way.

One way to be mindful of things that can turn up the dial on our emotions, or trigger us, is to plan. For example, if we know we have difficulty in math that causes us to have anxiety, and there is a math test on Thursday, we can plan for that emotion and have something to do to stay in control. If we know that when we change classes for 3rd period and we have to pass a certain student that causes problems for us, we can make a plan on how we can manage that situation ahead of time and keep our emotions under control.

**Reminder:** This is a great time to remember how we can encourage ourselves by thinking positive thoughts. You could think, "I am in control of my emotions," or other phrases to help you stay calm and think before you act. Add phrases to think about in your planner.

**Activity:** Look at the following list below and write them in the blue columns below based on whether it is something you DO control or something you DO NOT control.

| | |
|---|---|
| 1) Your height | 5) An F on a test |
| 2) What you eat for dinner | 6) The time you go to bed |
| 3) Your grades | 7) How many tasks you can accomplish in a day |
| 4) The mood of your teacher | 8) For how long you exercise |

| IN OUR CONTROL | NOT IN OUR CONTROL |
|---|---|
| | |

**Practice:** As you go through your day, remind yourself you are in control of your emotions and their intensity. You will get better at managing your emotions as you practice.

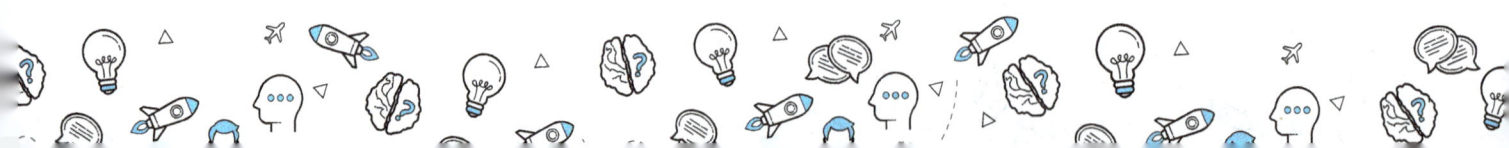

# Homework Log

Week beginning: ___ / ___ / ___

**My goal this week:** _____

_____

| | |
|---|---|
| **Monday**<br>___ / ___ | |
| **Tuesday**<br>___ / ___ | |
| **Wednesday**<br>___ / ___ | |
| **Thursday**<br>___ / ___ | |
| **Friday**<br>___ / ___ | |
| **Home/School Communication** | |

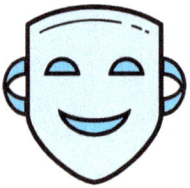

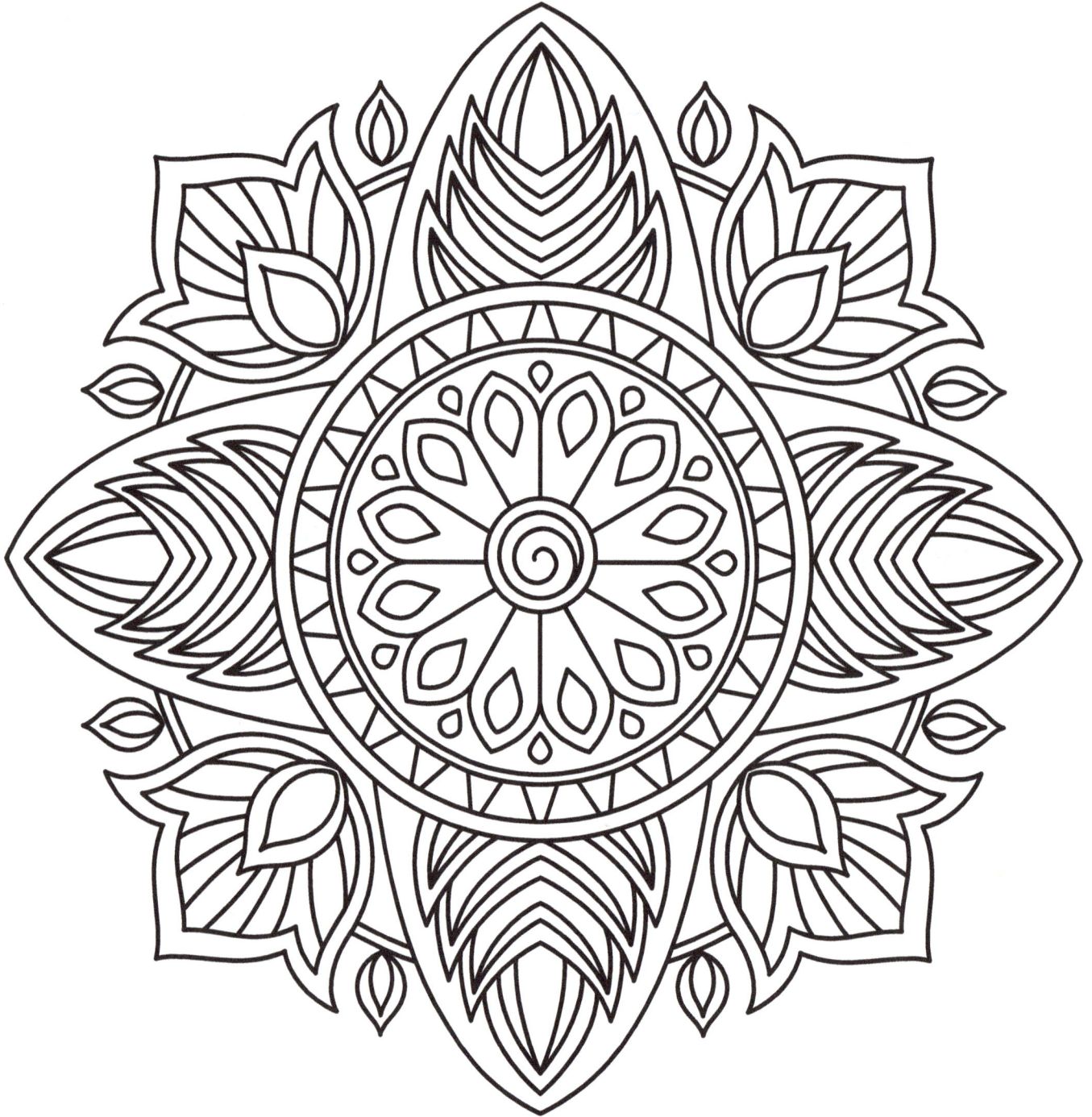

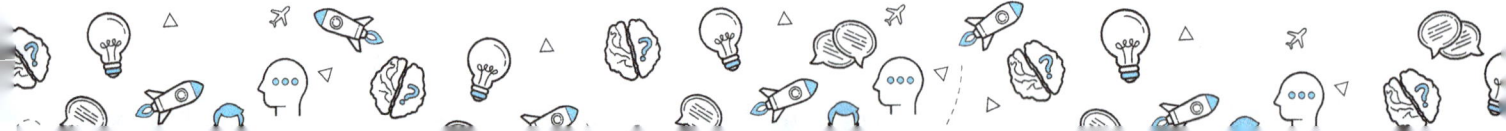

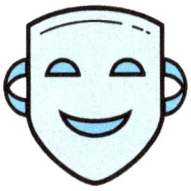

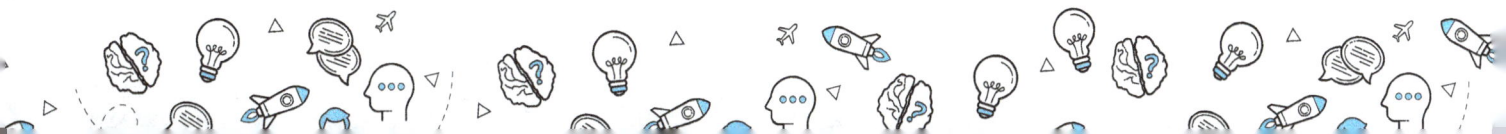

# The Great Big Mix

Mixed emotions happen when we experience more than one emotion at a time that are opposites. Think 'on' and 'off,' 'open' and 'closed,' 'up' and 'down' happening at the same time.

When we have negative emotions and a positive emotion at the same time, we can learn to accept the negative emotion and the feelings we have by focusing on the positive emotion that is also happening. Being able to deal with mixed emotions is a sign of maturity, and it shows that you are using more information about yourself, others, or situations to help you cope well through that event.

**Activity:** Talk through these mixed emotional experiences with a friend, teacher, or your family, so you are better prepared to handle situations in the future.

*Your dad got a new job after being out of work for a few months, but it means your family has to move.*

Emotions you may feel: _____ and _____

It's ok to feel _____, but I will focus on feeling _____ because _____.

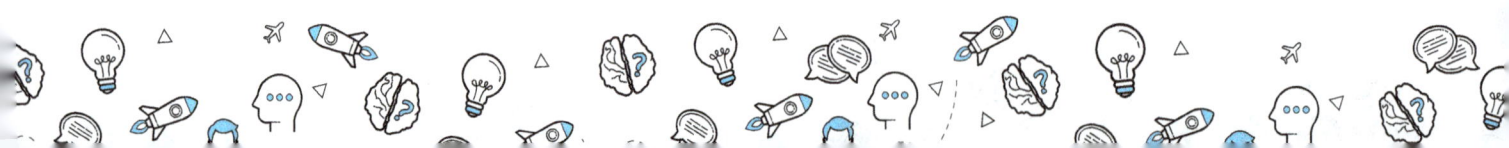

*You found a stray dog and took care of him for a week, and now his owner is coming to pick him up.*

Emotions you may feel: _____ and _____

It's ok to feel _____, but I will focus on feeling _____ because _____.

*You found some money in the parking lot when no one was around. Later you hear someone say that they lost the same amount of money that morning.*

Emotions you may feel: _____ and _____

It's ok to feel _____, but I will focus on feeling _____ because _____.

*You made the team, but your best friend did not.*

Emotions you may feel: _____ and _____

It's ok to feel _____, but I will focus on feeling _____ because _____.

*Your older sister enlisted in the military and will be learning to become a pilot like she always wanted to, but she will be leaving soon, and you will not see her for several months.*

Emotions you may feel: _____ and _____

It's ok to feel _____, but I will focus on feeling _____ because _____.

# Homework Log

Week beginning: ___ / ___ / ___

**My goal this week:** _____

_____

| | |
|---|---|
| **Monday** ___ / ___ | |
| **Tuesday** ___ / ___ | |
| **Wednesday** ___ / ___ | |
| **Thursday** ___ / ___ | |
| **Friday** ___ / ___ | |
| **Home/School Communication** | |

# Locus of Control

There are two extremes to locus of control - External, where people feel that others strongly influence what happens to them, and Internal, where people feel they are mostly responsible for things that happen to them. Students who feel they are successful based on their own effort and work have an Internal Locus of Control (LOC). Students who feel their success is more due to luck, fate, timing have an External Locus of Control (LOC).

Let's say you get picked to be on a team, or you are voted in as a leader at school or organization. If you have an Internal LOC, you will probably feel you deserve it because of your hard work, the quality of your character, or your personal effort. If you have an External LOC, you may feel that you achieved this success due to being lucky, etc.

What about something that happens that is negative? Let's say you lost at the tournament, failed a test, or did not get selected for something you wanted. If your LOC is internal, you may feel you are a failure, you may blame yourself, and you may criticize and get down on yourself and your qualities or attributes. As someone who has an external LOC, you may blame another person, blame favoritism by the coach, blame your parents for not doing something for you, etc.

**Activity:** Fill in the chart below and describe four situations that have happened to you. Did you respond with an external or internal LOC?

| | |
|---|---|
| **I felt:**<br><br>External ----------------------------------- Internal | **When:** |
| **I felt:**<br><br>External ----------------------------------- Internal | **When:** |
| **I felt:**<br><br>External ----------------------------------- Internal | **When:** |
| **I felt:**<br><br>External ----------------------------------- Internal | **When:** |

**Practice:** It's essential to view the concept of locus of control as a continuum. People aren't 100% external or 100% internal; they fall somewhere along a continuum line, with a predisposition to one side or the other. Observe yourself this week and indicate where you fall on the continuum.

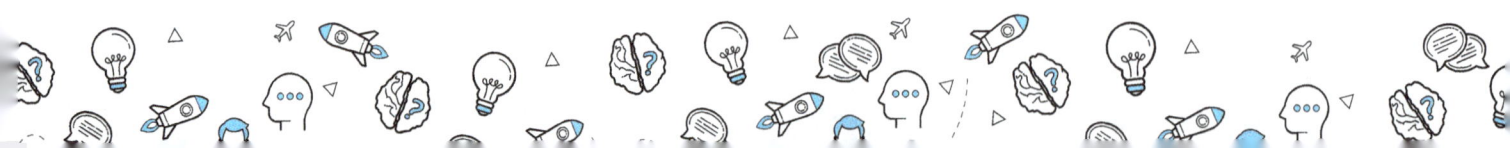

# Homework Log

Week beginning: ____ / ____ / ____

**My goal this week:** _____

_____

| | |
|---|---|
| **Monday** ___ / ___ | |
| **Tuesday** ___ / ___ | |
| **Wednesday** ___ / ___ | |
| **Thursday** ___ / ___ | |
| **Friday** ___ / ___ | |
| **Home/School Communication** | |

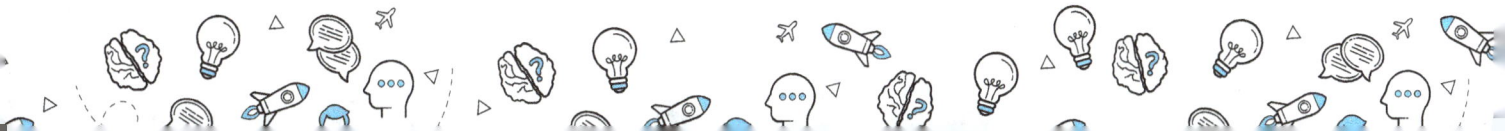

# I Have a Feeling That's Really a Need

Connection, physical well-being, safety, truth, enjoyment, peace, the ability to make decisions for yourself, and the need to be understood are needs we all have (paraphrased from the Center for Nonviolent Communication). We can have negative emotions and feelings when one or more of these needs are not being met. Once we can identify a need that we have, we can use that information to make changes or ask for help. For example, we become upset when others around us are not getting along.

**Why does that bother us?**

We have a need for harmony or peace in our lives.
We may not know why others are not getting along, and that bothers us.
We have a need for our community (people in our environment) to be close.
And, we have a need for safety and security in our relationships.

> **Reminder:** Just like situations and events that we know will happen, like a math test on Thursday, we can look at our environment and situations around us that affect our emotions and make a plan on how we respond.
>
> **Activity:** The Center for Nonviolent Communication has put together a process that starts with observing the situation, identifying your feelings, and then identifying your need. After we identify what we need, we can then ask questions or ask for help. Follow this process in these examples.

*Observation: I always struggle in math class, and tonight I just don't understand my math homework at all. I don't think I can do the homework; I'll turn in a blank piece of paper.*

Feelings:_____ Needs: _____ Request: _____

*Observation: My best friend is gossiping to me about one of my other friends. I think I might be getting in the middle of my two friends, and I'm not sure what to do.*

Feelings:_____ Needs: _____ Request: _____

*Observation: My friend and I had a long argument.*

Feelings:_____ Needs: _____ Request: _____

*Observation: I have a lot of homework, and my mom needs me to do some chores for her. I have not had a chance to watch TV or go outside with my friends.*

Feelings:_____ Needs: _____ Request: _____

> **Hint:** When making a request, ask in a way that is positive and polite. State what you are feeling, and what you need, and ask if the other person can help you.

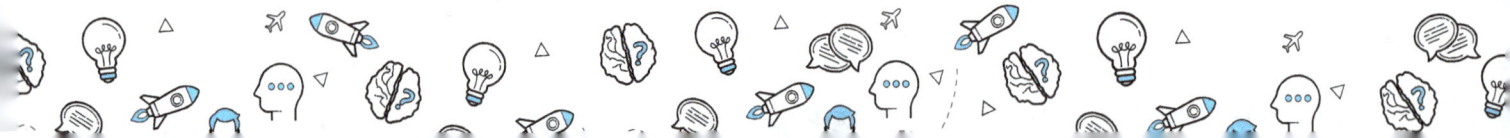

# Homework Log

Week beginning: ___ / ___ / ___

**My goal this week:** _____

_____

| | |
|---|---|
| **Monday** ___ / ___ | _____ <br> _____ <br> _____ <br> _____ |
| **Tuesday** ___ / ___ | _____ <br> _____ <br> _____ <br> _____ |
| **Wednesday** ___ / ___ | _____ <br> _____ <br> _____ <br> _____ |
| **Thursday** ___ / ___ | _____ <br> _____ <br> _____ <br> _____ |
| **Friday** ___ / ___ | _____ <br> _____ <br> _____ <br> _____ |
| **Home/School Communication** | |

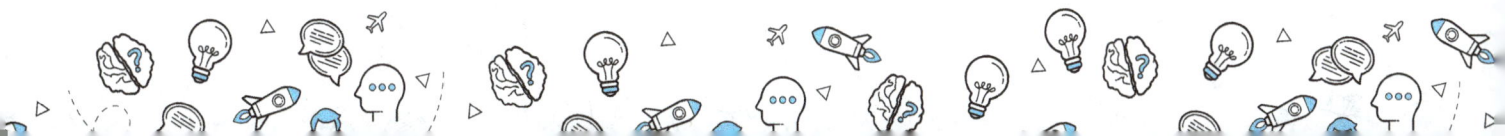

# Keep Growing

Now that you are in 7th grade, you are probably facing more situations that may case you stress and it is important to also grow more tools to address stress. There are more classes and teachers, there are only about 5 minutes to get to the next class, and there are new social situations. For some students, the hallways and classrooms can feel more like a battle zone than a safe place. Emotions are more intense, how important the opinions of others can seem, students feel left out, and many are teased. These situations can make you feel like nothing will ever get better.

Research shows that students who spend time learning to change their thoughts improved their ability to deal with stressful situations, stayed calm, and had a better outlook. How did they do this? They learned to turn their thoughts around, to bend their brains, and think about their situations in a completely different way. Students who thought they were being left out of something, learned that it did not mean something was wrong with them.

Students who can think that the work may be hard to do, but they know they need to learn the information have the point of view that the glass is half full, and they can work to fill it up. They may not always be successful, but they try. Through their effort, they learn, and their glass gets a little fuller than before. This is called having a "growth mindset." It is a frame of mind that looks at what is possible, looks at setbacks as temporary and not the end of the world, and takes challenges as opportunities.

**Activity:** Take the fixed mindset thoughts and change them to show growth mindset.

| FIXED MINDSET | GROWTH MINDSET |
|---|---|
| I'll never be that pretty/handsome. | |
| This teacher hates me. | |
| I have too much work to do. I can't do all this homework! | |
| Coach never puts me in the game. I'll never be good enough for him/her. I should just quit. | |
| All the books my English teacher assigns are boring. How will I ever get through this new novel? | |

**Remember:** "Obstacles don't have to stop you. If you run into a wall, don't turn around and give up. Figure out how to climb it, go through it, or work around it." - *Michael Jordan*

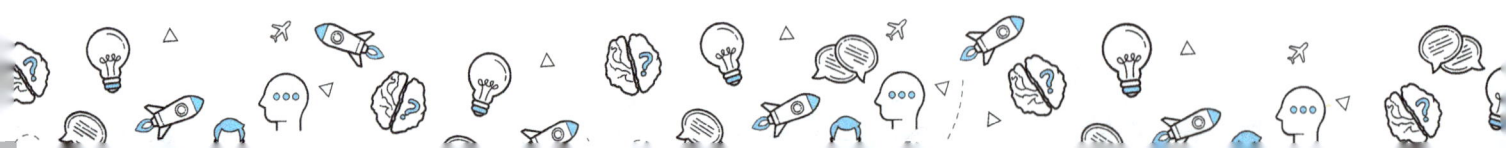

# Homework Log

Week beginning: ____ / ____ / ____

**My goal this week:** _____

_____

| | |
|---|---|
| **Monday** <br> ___ / ___ | _____ <br> _____ <br> _____ <br> _____ |
| **Tuesday** <br> ___ / ___ | _____ <br> _____ <br> _____ <br> _____ |
| **Wednesday** <br> ___ / ___ | _____ <br> _____ <br> _____ <br> _____ |
| **Thursday** <br> ___ / ___ | _____ <br> _____ <br> _____ |
| **Friday** <br> ___ / ___ | _____ <br> _____ <br> _____ <br> _____ |
| **Home/School Communication** | |

# REVIEW WEEK! Small Wins Make a Big Impact

Take some time this week to reflect and observe yourself, your emotions, your responses and reactions. How are you doing? Be mindful, present and focused as you answer these reflections:

What did you learn about yourself over the past 9 weeks? Describe yourself:

I am _____

I can _____

I am _____

I have _____

I am _____

I will _____

I am _____

I want _____

I am _____

Describe something positive you have noticed about yourself since the start of school:

_____

_____

_____

Reflect on your goals you made for this year. Have you started working on your goals? How are you doing?

_____

_____

_____

**Remember:** Small steps are still steps forward. If you have not achieved your goal, or you have not noticed changes yet, that is ok. Change is a process, and we are always learning.

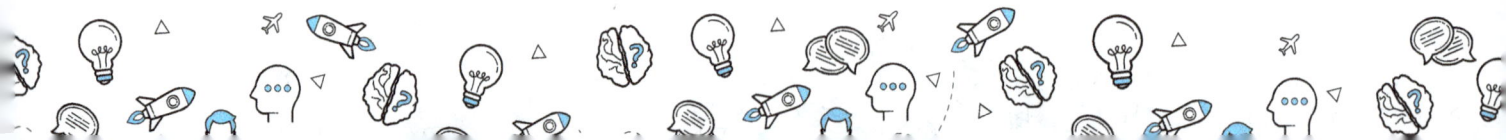

# Homework Log

Week beginning: ___ / ___ / ___

My goal this week: _____

_____

| | |
|---|---|
| **Monday**<br>___ / ___ | _____<br>_____<br>_____ |
| **Tuesday**<br>___ / ___ | _____<br>_____<br>_____ |
| **Wednesday**<br>___ / ___ | _____<br>_____<br>_____<br>_____ |
| **Thursday**<br>___ / ___ | _____<br>_____<br>_____ |
| **Friday**<br>___ / ___ | _____<br>_____<br>_____ |
| **Home/School Communication** | |

# 10 Week Goal Check-In

Look back at the goals you set for yourself at the beginning of the year. Add notes to check-in or make changes to your goals. It's ok to add or change your goals a little, but keep pushing yourself to grow this year. If you feel you have met your goal, make a new goal for yourself at the bottom of this page.

| | How I'm doing on this goal: | What I need to adjust or continue working on: |
|---|---|---|
| Goal: | | |
| Goal: | | |
| Goal: | | |
| Goal: | | |
| Goal: | | |

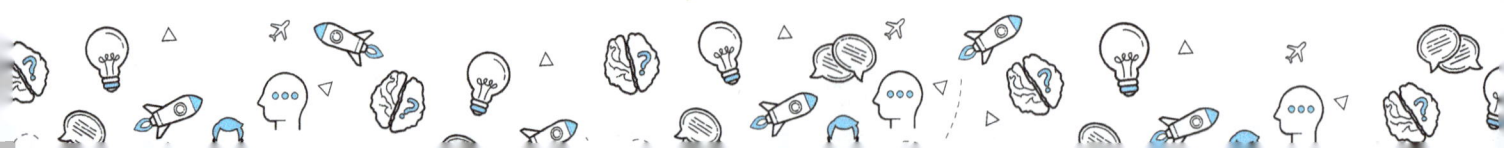

# Social-Emotional Learning Connection

Think about a story, show, movie, song, or social media post you have read or watched over the past 10 weeks that connects to the learning about self-awareness.

What was the source called? _____

How does this text connect to self-awareness and social-emotional learning? Draw a picture or write your answer below.

What was it that made you think about self-awareness? What did you learn about self-awareness from this source?

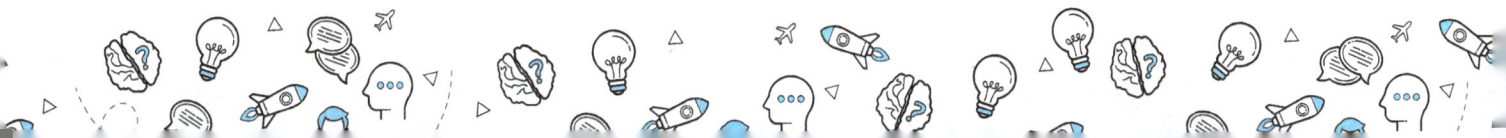

_____

_____

_____

_____

_____

_____

_____

_____

# Notes

# Notes

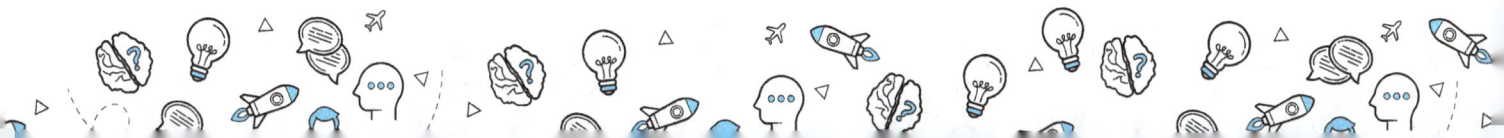

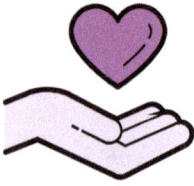

# Courage and Kindness

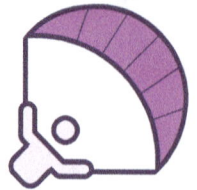

You have just finished the theme on identity and mindset, and we are now transitioning to courage and kindness with a focus on the social-emotional competency of relationship skills.

**Throughout this theme, you will be focusing on:**

1) Developing and maintaining healthy relationships (Relationship-building)
2) Peer pressure, bullying, and boundaries (Communication)
3) Compassion and empathy (Social engagement & Teamwork)
4) Resiliency and seeking help (Communication & Relationship-building)

Showing kindness to others, and building quality relationships with your family and friends are important. Learn more about the qualities of courage and kindness these next ten weeks by completing the activities below. You will get to read, listen to, and taste new things to help you experience courage & kindness.

**Read:** From your school or community library, check out *The Boy at the Back of the Class* by Onjali Q. Rauf. Both kindness and courage are displayed in this book about a Syrian refugee who comes to England and is new to the class.

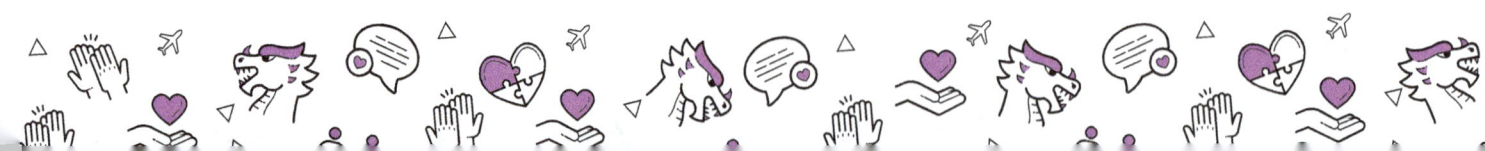

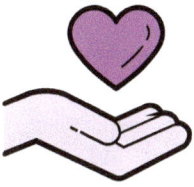

# Courage and Kindness

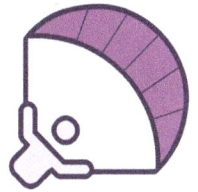

**Listen to:** With your carer's permission, go online to listen to "Count on Me" by Bruno Mars. Mars sings about friendships. How does he describe friendship?

What are some of the kind acts Bruno Mars describes in this song? _____

_____

_____

What is your favorite line or part of this song? _____

_____

_____

How are you a friend to someone else with the characteristics described in this song? _____

_____

_____

**Taste:** Some foods you will never like, but you don't know if you don't like them if you don't try them! Try something you haven't ever tasted before -- either something you have at home or go to the grocery store and try a new-to-you food. Give your taste buds a chance to really taste it by trying several bites. Be courageous! You might be about to find out your new favorite food.

The new food I tried was _____

It tasted _____

_____

How did it feel to be courageous and try something new? _____

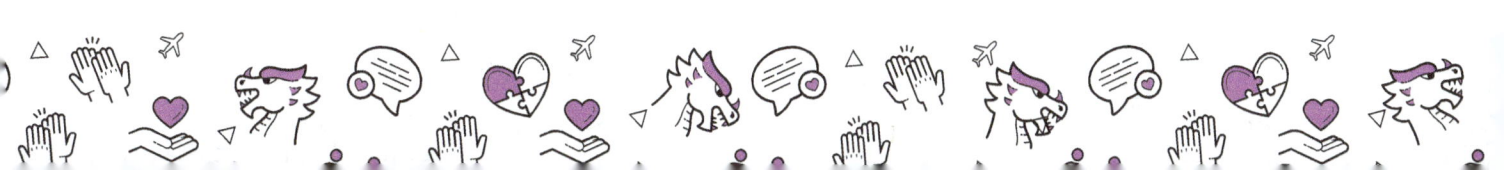

_____

# Let's Be Friends

Friendship is a mysterious thing. If you look around, you will find people who are friends who share lots of similarities. You can just as quickly find friends who seem to be complete opposites. So, what is it that makes people friends? One friendship that celebrates differences is the friendship between Dwayne "The Rock" Johnson and Kevin Hart. They tease each other about their differences in size, food, and interests. But the public gets a sense of their deep friendship, especially when Kevin Hart was seriously injured in a car accident. Afterward, Kevin was encouraged to work hard to recover by his bodybuilding friend, Dwayne. Although they have noticeable differences, they said in an interview that what made them such good friends was they had so much fun together. As time went on, they became "like brothers."

When trying to make a friend, it is important to identify others who have similar interests and values as you. Some things may be non-negotiable in a friend, such as always having your back. These qualities might be something you need to think about. As you think about what is important to you in a friend, you are probably identifying the type of friend you would be.

**Activity:** Fill out the following boxes to help you reflect on your friendships.

| Things I need in a friend: | My non-negotiables in a friend: |
|---|---|
| | |
| Qualities I bring to a friendship: | To me, friendship is: |
| | |

**Reminder:** There are different types of friends. Some will be friends in certain classes or situations and will be people that you get along with, can talk to, and maybe text. Others may be more like acquaintances; you know who they are, and you can say 'hello,' but you do not really talk. Close friends, like The Rock and Kevin Hart, are few and may take time to find.

# Homework Log

Week beginning: ___ / ___ / ___

**My goal this week:** _____
_____

| | |
|---|---|
| **Monday** ___ / ___ | |
| **Tuesday** ___ / ___ | |
| **Wednesday** ___ / ___ | |
| **Thursday** ___ / ___ | |
| **Friday** ___ / ___ | |
| **Home/School Communication** | |

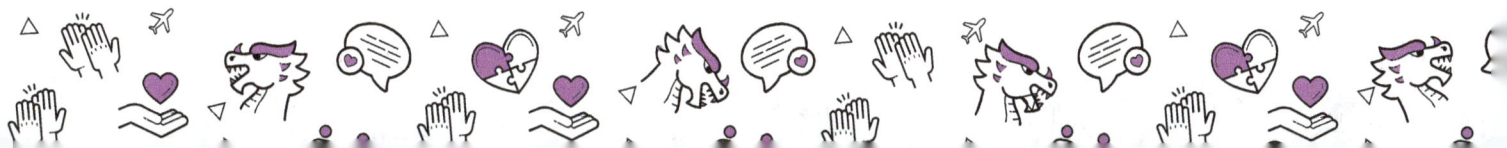

# Connections and Relationships

There are different types of relationships. Friends are people you are close to, talk to often, and share your thoughts with. You also have friends who are more like acquaintances; you know who they are, and you say 'hello,' but you do not really share deeply. As you meet people and make connections, you build community with others. As you go through this year, and in the future, these connections of people may be sources of help, comfort, support, or may develop into good friends or a close friendship.

To make good connections that could possibly develop into a friendship, specific skills are needed. The first is knowing how to have a conversation with others. Start a conversation by asking questions, noticing something about the other person. Extend the conversation by asking questions, asking for more information or details, and sharing your own experience. People want to know we are listening, so focus on what they are saying and do not take over the conversation.

Making a broad group of acquaintances and friends broadens your world. Having a group of different points of view, different areas of interest, all add to your store of knowledge and make you more well rounded.

**Activity:** Share your friendship story! Tell about how you made a connection that became a friend. How did you meet? What did you talk about? What did you have in common? What were your differences?

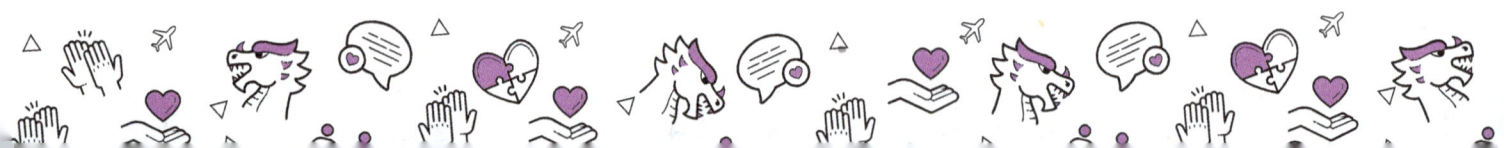

_____

_____

_____

_____

_____

_____

_____

_____

_____

_____

# Homework Log

Week beginning: ____ / ____ / ____

My goal this week: _____

_____

| | |
|---|---|
| **Monday**<br>___ / ___ | _____<br>_____<br>_____<br>_____ |
| **Tuesday**<br>___ / ___ | _____<br>_____<br>_____<br>_____ |
| **Wednesday**<br>___ / ___ | _____<br>_____<br>_____<br>_____ |
| **Thursday**<br>___ / ___ | _____<br>_____<br>_____<br>_____ |
| **Friday**<br>___ / ___ | _____<br>_____<br>_____<br>_____ |
| **Home/School Communication** | |

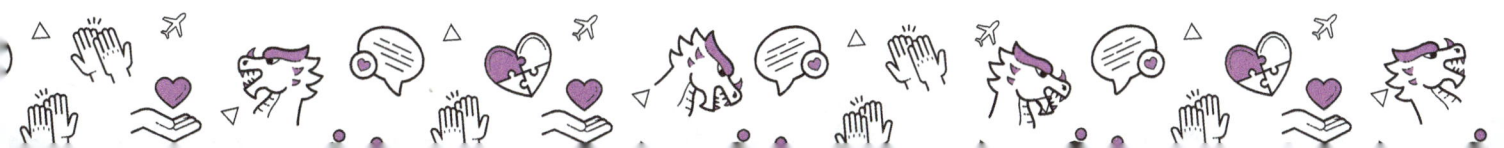

# Protective Boundaries

You likely have felt pressure to do things by "friends" that you do not want to do, or you think it is not right to do. Often this happens when we are with a group of people because it is easier for multiple people to get someone to do something they do not necessarily want to do. It may be hard to recognize this is happening because we want to fit in and be part of the group. Many times, these are people we think we want to be friends with, we want to impress, so we go along with their ideas instead of remembering our values and who we are.

You may have had a situation where you have a good friend who seems like the perfect friend; you enjoy their company, you like a lot of the same things, they make you laugh. Then one day, that friend can do something that we do not expect, which can change the relationship. They may try and pressure you to join what they are doing and tell you that you are not a friend if you don't. You may hear that they won't be your friend anymore, or you may feel you will lose their friendship if you don't join in.

When students give into doing things they do not want to do or allow things to happen they do not agree with, and they let go of their values and identity, they are giving in to peer pressure. As difficult as it may seem to understand, the people who would uncomfortably pressure you are not true friends. It is important to know our identity and our values because then we know our boundaries.

**Activity:** Answer the following questions to start defining your protective boundaries.

What types of things, actions, or words, would be uncomfortable for you to take part in?

_____

_____

What negative qualities would you avoid having in a "friend" because they may negatively influence you?

_____

_____

❝ *Give, but do not allow yourself to be used. Love, but do not allow your heart to be abused. Trust, but do not be naive. Listen to others, but do not lose yourself. … Boundaries are part of self-care. They are healthy, normal and necessary"* **– Doreen Virtue** ❞

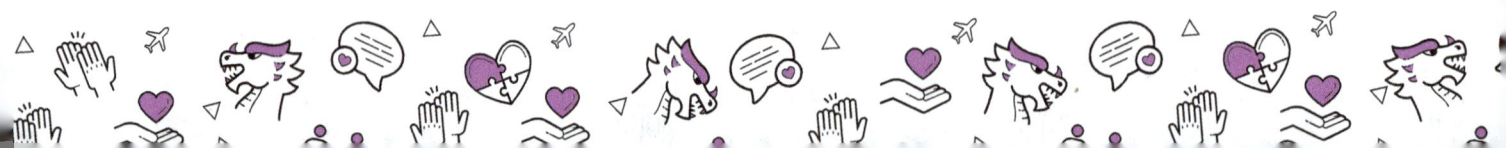

# Homework Log

Week beginning: ___ / ___ / ___

**My goal this week:** _____

_____

| | |
|---|---|
| **Monday**<br>___ / ___ | _____<br>_____<br>_____<br>_____ |
| **Tuesday**<br>___ / ___ | _____<br>_____<br>_____ |
| **Wednesday**<br>___ / ___ | _____<br>_____<br>_____ |
| **Thursday**<br>___ / ___ | _____<br>_____<br>_____ |
| **Friday**<br>___ / ___ | _____<br>_____<br>_____ |
| **Home/School Communication** | |

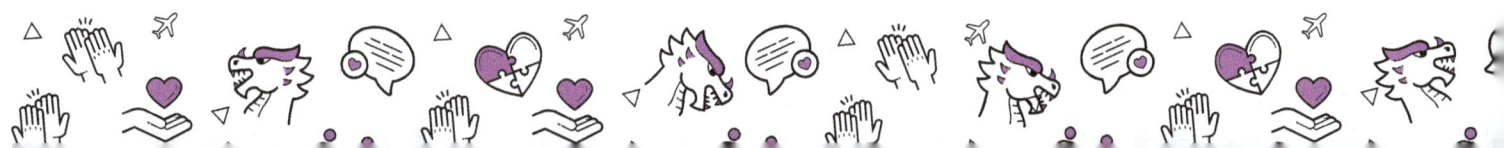

# Be Kind, Rewind

Many times when you have so many things to manage, it is hard to maintain a consistent focus. You may start to lose focus on one area, like studying because your activities or responsibilities take a lot of your attention. When you lose focus and make a bad grade or miss out on something, you can be disappointed. As much as you may strive to meet your goals you created at the beginning of the year, there may be setbacks. It is important to know that everyone experiences setbacks and disappointments.

When you have negative feelings related to your performance in school, an activity, or in your relationships with others, it is time to be kind to yourself. Your identity, remember, is not the grade on your report card, or the people you hang out with. Remember to give yourself a break whenever disappointments happen and learn from those situations. Go back, rewind, and look at how you defined yourself as a student and as a person.

**Activity:** Everyone has negative feelings at times when things don't go how we planned or hoped. Change your frame of mind, feelings, mindset, and show kindness to yourself, by doing the following:

Visualize:
- Take a deep breath and blow out your breath slowly. Do this a few times.
- Close your eyes and think about something you did that was good, helpful, or kind.
- Picture those memories in your mind.
- Remember how you felt when you had those experiences.

Get Active:
- Take a break and do something that makes you feel good, like playing a sport you like, playing music, or spending time with your friends or family.

Reflect and Learn:
- When you have a disappointing experience, stop and think about what you have learned from it. What can you try next time? What can you do differently?

Positive Mindset:
- Instead of thinking about something that did not go right, think about things you are good at, things you do well. Picture those things and remember how you felt when you took part in those activities.

66 *Be yourself; everyone else is already taken.* – **Oscar Wilde** 99

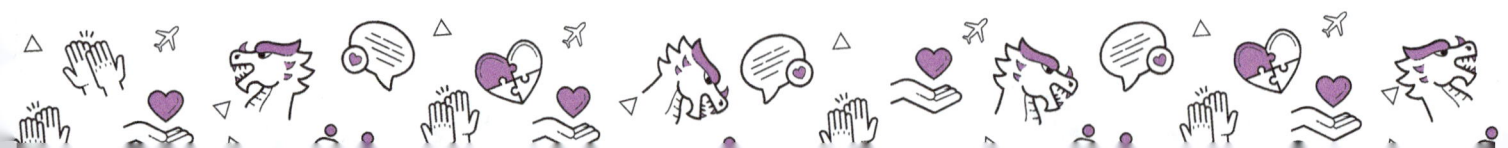

# Homework Log

Week beginning: ____ / ____ / ____

**My goal this week:** _____

_____

| | |
|---|---|
| **Monday**<br>___ / ___ | _____<br>_____<br>_____<br>_____ |
| **Tuesday**<br>___ / ___ | _____<br>_____<br>_____ |
| **Wednesday**<br>___ / ___ | _____<br>_____<br>_____<br>_____ |
| **Thursday**<br>___ / ___ | _____<br>_____<br>_____ |
| **Friday**<br>___ / ___ | _____<br>_____<br>_____<br>_____ |
| **Home/School Communication** | |

# Sympathy and Empathy

If feelings were a video game, empathy would be a level up above sympathy. Sympathy is the act of, or the ability to share the feelings of another. Sympathy cards, hugs, and affection, providing a meal to others, are all ways we express sympathy. Showing sympathy can indicate that we identify what others are feeling, and we want them to feel better. Sympathy is great, and an expected response to most situations where others around us are feeling sad, discouraged, or upset.

Empathy is the act of understanding and experiencing the feelings, thoughts, and experiences of someone else. You do not need to know the person to have empathy. For example, when you read a book, you can have empathy for a character, and share the same feelings of the characters you are reading about.

Most people have a good understanding of sympathy. Empathy is a little different because empathy is understanding at some level the emotions of others. When we show empathy, or we are empathetic, we listen to others, we do not show judgment or try to give advice, and we are accepting of their feelings. Empathy helps us treat people we care about how they want to be treated. Empathy helps us understand the needs of others. We can communicate better when we show empathy.

Some actions that show you are sensitive to other's feelings are letting someone go first, or letting someone have something you want because they need it more than you. When you show empathy to someone, you may experience the same feelings that they do. You may also feel good to be able to relate to someone else and help them through something upsetting to them.

**Reminder:** All our work at the beginning of the year in understanding feelings and emotions is essential so you can recognize the feelings and emotions of others and show empathy for others.

**Activity:** Talk about these scenarios with a friend or family, and discuss how you would handle these situations with empathy rather than getting upset or angry.

- You get into an argument with a friend because they want to borrow your phone charger again. This is happening a lot and starting to get on your nerves.
- Your sibling is having a bad day and is yelling at everyone, including you.
- Your friend invites you over but does not invite your other friend who is standing next to you when she asks you to come over.

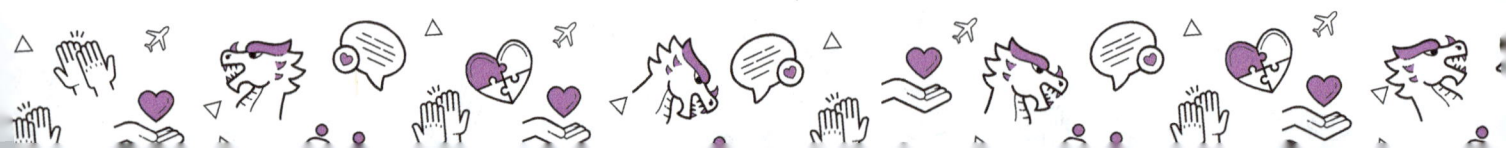

# Homework Log

Week beginning: ____ / ____ / ____

**My goal this week:** _____

_____

| | |
|---|---|
| **Monday** ___ / ___ | |
| **Tuesday** ___ / ___ | |
| **Wednesday** ___ / ___ | |
| **Thursday** ___ / ___ | |
| **Friday** ___ / ___ | |
| **Home/School Communication** | |

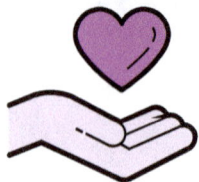

# COLORING

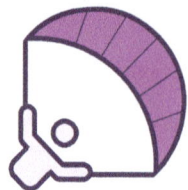

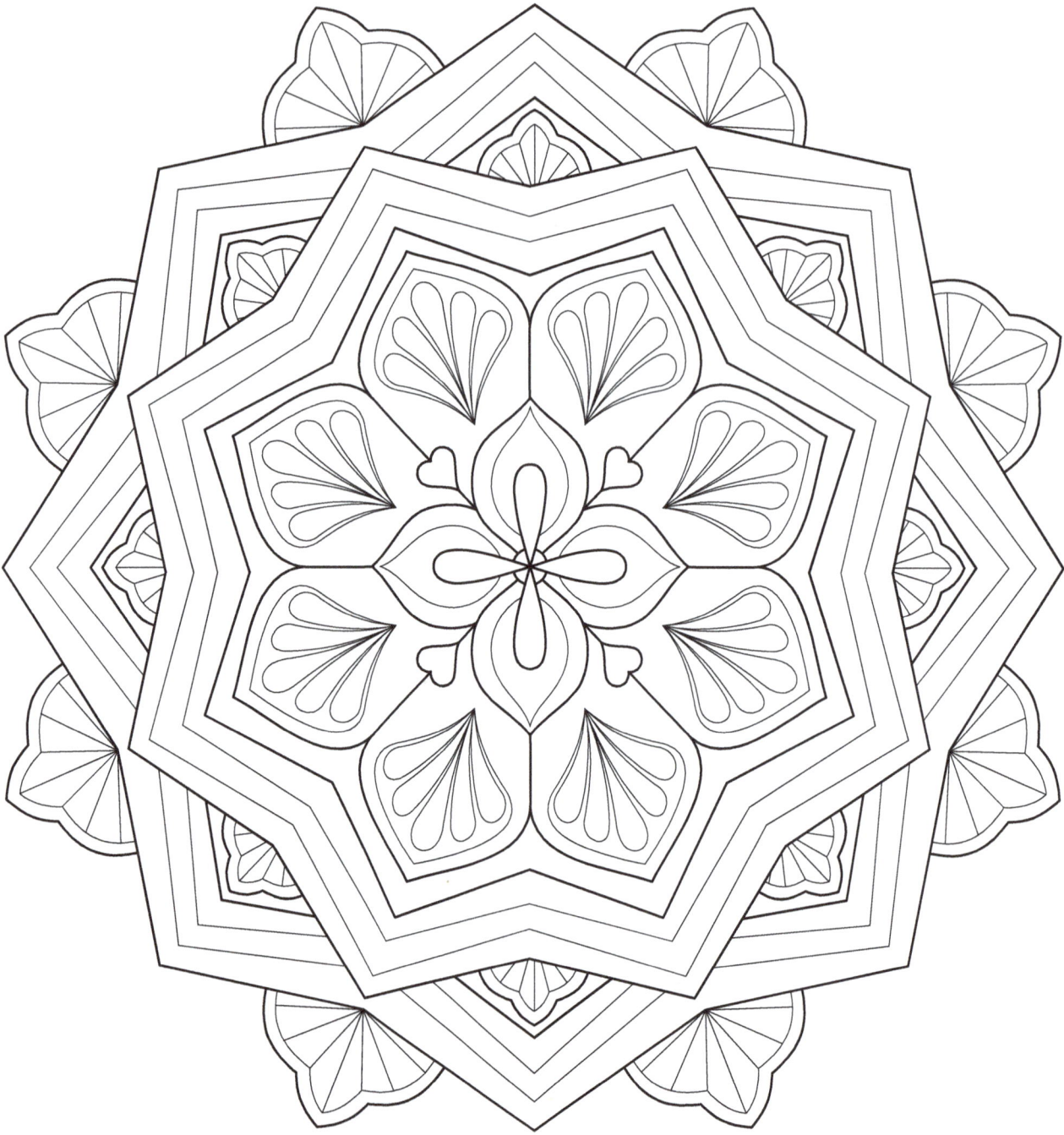

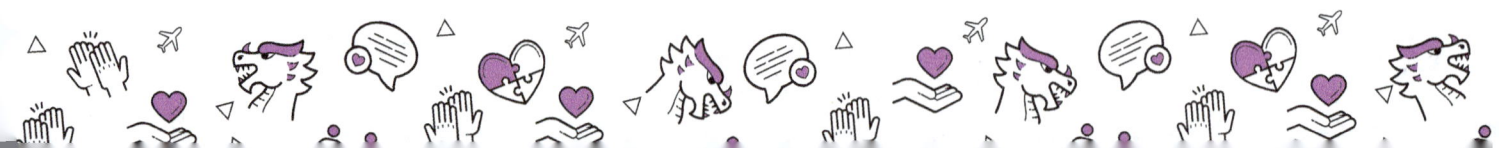

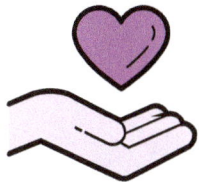

# DOODLING PAGE

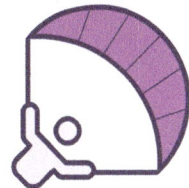

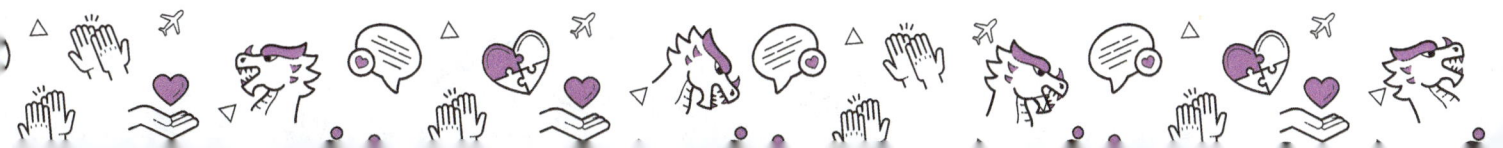

# Let's Be Blunt

Bullying is a repeated, harmful, and unwanted action toward another person. There is usually an imbalance of power between the bully and the victim; for example, the bully is older, bigger, or someone of influence. Bullying takes many forms. Popular forms of bullying are name-calling, aggressive teasing, racial comments, aggressive or persistent sarcasm, rumors, and intimidation. Bullying can be physical, such as unwanted touching, hitting, spitting, tripping, pushing, or other aggressive acts with objects. Bullying can be social and involve groups such as excluding someone, humiliating someone in public, or put-downs in front of others. Today more than ever is the threat of cyberbullying, which is like verbal bullying but is through social media or texts.

**There are steps you need to take if you are being bullied:**

1) Tell someone you trust. If you don't feel comfortable telling an adult, start by confiding in a friend with a goal of talking to an adult about it.
2) Report! Reporting is sharing legitimate information to protect yourself or another person.
3) Know there are laws designed to address bullying.
4) Know you have the right to speak up for yourself and let an adult know what you need to feel safe.
5) Document, block, and report. Take pictures to document actions or words used. Block the person on social media. Report to adults.
6) Be your own advocate and make a Self Action Plan using this national resource: https://pacerteensagainstbullying.org/advocacy-for-self/%20student-action-plan/.

**Activity:** Statistics show that bullying is happening more than we realize. The effects of bullying are long-lasting and traumatic. Find out about the experiences of others and take a survey of 20 people in your school to find out more about bullying. Here are some suggested questions for your survey:

| Have you been bullied at school? | What happened? |
|---|---|

| Have you been bullied outside of school? | How did you feel when that happened? |
|---|---|

| How did you feel when that happened? | How did you stop it? |
|---|---|

Discuss your survey with your class and family.

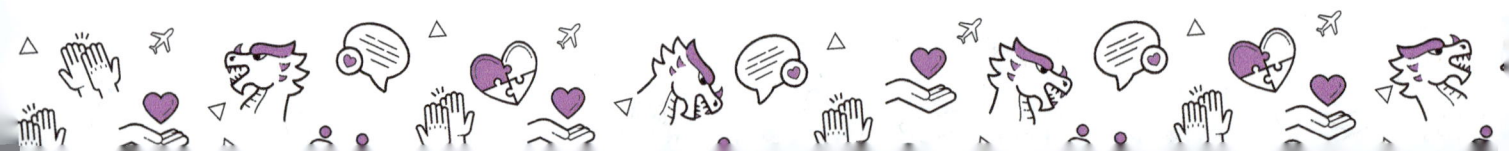

# Homework Log

Week beginning: ____ / ____ / ____

**My goal this week:** _____

_____

| | |
|---|---|
| **Monday** ___ / ___ | |
| **Tuesday** ___ / ___ | |
| **Wednesday** ___ / ___ | |
| **Thursday** ___ / ___ | |
| **Friday** ___ / ___ | |
| **Home/School Communication** | |

# Keep Bouncing

You have probably played basketball, or at least bounced a ball. Often PE teachers have a large bin of basketballs, and students may pick through the balls to find one that is the fullest and has the best bounce. The balls that have lost some air are a little squishy and can barely bounce; they fall flat. Resilience is how balls bounce back from being pushed down to the floor. You can also see differences in the resilience of the basketball depending on how hard you bounce it; the harder you push it to the ground, the higher it will bounce up into the air.

Although we are not basketballs, people are also resilient. We have stress and pressure that pushes us down sometimes; peer pressure, homework, teacher's expectations, parent's expectations, and the pressure we put on ourselves to reach our personal goals. Some people can feel pushed down by other people's situations around us that we empathize with.

The sense of pressure may be building up more than your past experiences. With every new year comes new opportunities to do new things where you may succeed, or experience disappointment. It is in these low times that research says gives us the most important chances to learn about ourselves.

**Reminder:** Instead of air in a basketball, people have grit that gives us the ability to bounce back when we have a problem. Grit is the firmness of mind or spirit. Just like a firm basketball can bounce well and bounce high, people with a lot of grit will be resilient enough in their minds and their inner self to not let the pressures of life made them fall flat.

**Activity:** In this activity, you are going to rate yourself on a scale of 1 to 5, with 1 being low and 5 being great on elements of resilience skills or abilities. It is important to assess how well you do in these areas to know what you need to work on to build up your resilience or get some grit.

_____ I have support from other people in my life.

_____ I can accept myself for who I really am.

_____ I have confidence in my ability to cope with adversity.

_____ I am good at communicating and interacting with others in times of stress.

_____ I am good at facing challenging problems in life and solving them.

_____ I can cope with my emotions when there is a problem.

_____ **Total**

What is your total score? What areas were lower? What made you give yourself that score? What can you do to improve in that area to get a higher score?

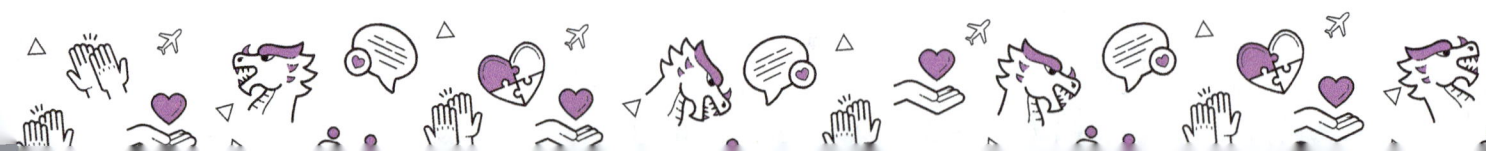

# Homework Log

**My goal this week:** _____

_____

| | |
|---|---|
| **Monday**<br>___ / ___ | _____<br>_____<br>_____<br>_____ |
| **Tuesday**<br>___ / ___ | _____<br>_____<br>_____ |
| **Wednesday**<br>___ / ___ | _____<br>_____<br>_____<br>_____ |
| **Thursday**<br>___ / ___ | _____<br>_____<br>_____ |
| **Friday**<br>___ / ___ | _____<br>_____<br>_____<br>_____ |
| **Home/School Communication** | |

# Help! I Need Somebody!

The Beatles song "Help" is about someone trying to do everything themselves, and over time, they realized they needed some help. The song says they may ask anyone to help them; maybe they did not know who to ask.

You may think being in 7th grade means being more independent, and you may feel you are on your own. Not true. Yes, people in your life may have new expectations for you, but no one wants you to be isolated. Asking for help is not a weakness; it does not signal that you are giving up.

Asking for help is a sign that you are smart enough to know that someone else may have an answer that you can use instead of having to figure it out on your own. If you know someone has discovered a way to do something, solve a problem, cope with setbacks, it makes sense to ask them to help you.

Asking for help can happen in different ways. You can talk to your teacher after class, or ask the teacher for an appointment. Find a friend who has the skills you need help with and ask them to help you. Be specific when asking for help. Saying you do not know how to do math is too general; saying you do not understand algebra question #3 is a much better way to ask for help.

**Reminder:** Asking for help is a way to develop grit and resilience.

**Activity:** Identify things you will need to ask for help. For example, a project where you have to make something, you have to go to the library, you don't understand a new skill that was taught and there is a test about it coming up. Use this technique all year in your planner.

| WHAT WILL I NEED HELP WITH? | WHO CAN I ASK? |
| --- | --- |
|  |  |
|  |  |
|  |  |
|  |  |

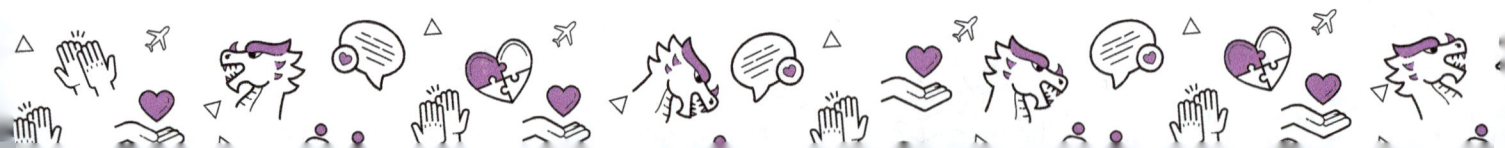

# Homework Log

**My goal this week:** _____

_____

| | |
|---|---|
| **Monday**<br>___ / ___ | _____<br>_____<br>_____<br>_____ |
| **Tuesday**<br>___ / ___ | _____<br>_____<br>_____<br>_____ |
| **Wednesday**<br>___ / ___ | _____<br>_____<br>_____<br>_____ |
| **Thursday**<br>___ / ___ | _____<br>_____<br>_____<br>_____ |
| **Friday**<br>___ / ___ | _____<br>_____<br>_____<br>_____ |
| **Home/School Communication** | |

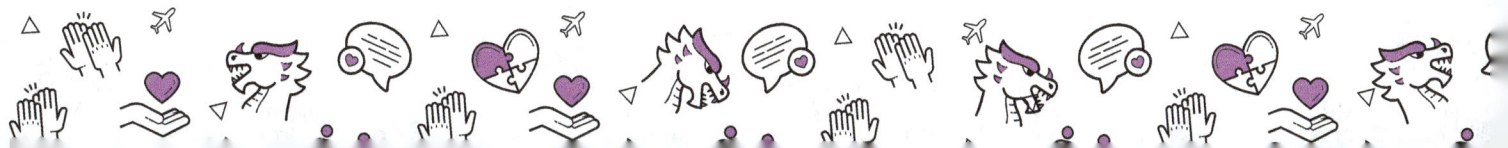

# I Have a Problem!

We are not talking about math here! We often have times where we are faced with a social problem, and we do not know what to do. Many times, we respond the same way to a problem no matter how serious or how big the problem is. We might lose a pencil, or can not find a paper as quickly as we want to, and our reaction is huge! We might yell out, get mad, hit the desk, or throw something. Looking back at our reactions, we can see how we sometimes overreact. Our big reactions can make a small problem seem to be worse than it actually is. Once we know what the problem is, how big the problem is, and the facts about the problem, we can respond better and solve the problem.

| HOW BIG IS THE PROBLEM, AND WHAT CAN I DO? | |
|---|---|
| 1) **Small** | The problem is not dangerous, will not last long, and may only affect me I can be calm, flexible, ignore minor problems. |
| 2) **Not that big** | The problem is not dangerous; it may last about 10 minutes, can be solved without help, may affect one other person and me. Fix the problem myself, be calm, and be flexible. |
| 3) **Medium** | The problem might need adult help, may last about a day, can be more challenging to solve, may affect a few more people and me. I need to tell an adult, stay calm, be patient, help as much as I can, and share my feelings if I am afraid or worried. |
| 4) **Big problem** | The problem may be dangerous, may last for a week, can be hard to solve, and can affect many people. I need to find an adult right away, be patient, help as much as I can, and share my feelings if I am afraid or worried. |
| 5) **Huge Serious Problem!** | The problem is very dangerous and is out of my control to solve. I need to listen to adults and follow directions, stay calm, be patient and flexible, help if I can, and share my feelings if I am afraid or worried. |

**Activity:** Brainstorm some of the problems you have had recently.

▸ How big was the problem?
▸ How did you solve the problem?
▸ What could be another, perhaps better, solution to your problem?

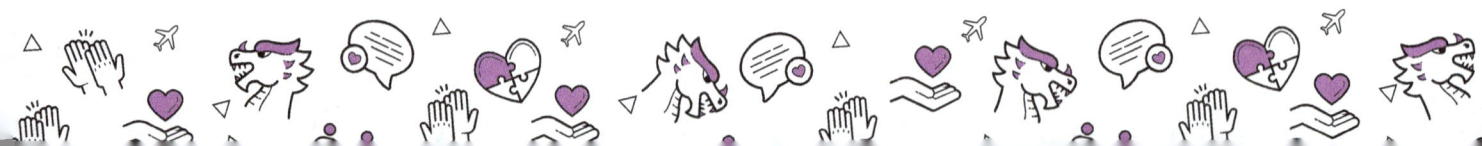

# Homework Log

Week beginning: ____ / ____ / ____

My goal this week: _____

_____

| | |
|---|---|
| **Monday** ___ / ___ | _____<br>_____<br>_____<br>_____ |
| **Tuesday** ___ / ___ | _____<br>_____<br>_____ |
| **Wednesday** ___ / ___ | _____<br>_____<br>_____<br>_____ |
| **Thursday** ___ / ___ | _____<br>_____<br>_____ |
| **Friday** ___ / ___ | _____<br>_____<br>_____<br>_____ |
| **Home/School Communication** | |

# It's Review Week! Balancing Our Connections

Over the past 9 weeks, you learned about making friendships, developing relationships and connections, creating healthy boundaries with people, and bullies. Often, the relationship we need to work on most is with ourselves. You focused on being kind to yourself, on your successes, doing hard things, and pushing yourself through difficult situations. You talked about being more independent, resilient, and asking for help. Taking time to understand our boundaries, recognizing what we need in a friend, knowing when to push ourselves not to give up, and when to ask for help all take time.

**Activity:** After learning some important information about yourself, reflect, and create a description of yourself. Think about your accomplishments this school year: what kind of boundaries you made for yourself, what qualities you demonstrate as a friend, and what qualities you look for in a friend. Describe how you show kindness to yourself and how you can get help when you need it.

_____

_____

_____

_____

_____

_____

_____

_____

_____

_____

_____

_____

_____

_____

_____

_____

_____

# Homework Log

Week beginning: ____ / ____ / ____

My goal this week: _____

_____

| | |
|---|---|
| **Monday**<br>___ / ___ | _____<br>_____<br>_____<br>_____ |
| **Tuesday**<br>___ / ___ | _____<br>_____<br>_____ |
| **Wednesday**<br>___ / ___ | _____<br>_____<br>_____<br>_____ |
| **Thursday**<br>___ / ___ | _____<br>_____<br>_____ |
| **Friday**<br>___ / ___ | _____<br>_____<br>_____<br>_____ |
| **Home/School Communication** | |

# 10 week Goal Check-In

Look back at the goals you set for yourself at the beginning of the year or at our last goal check-in. Add notes to check in or make changes to your goals. It's ok to add or change your goals a little, but keep pushing yourself to grow this year. If you feel you have met your goal, make a new goal for yourself at the bottom of this page.

| | How I'm doing on this goal: | What I need to adjust or continue working on: |
|---|---|---|
| Goal: | | |
| Goal: | | |
| Goal: | | |
| Goal: | | |
| Goal: | | |

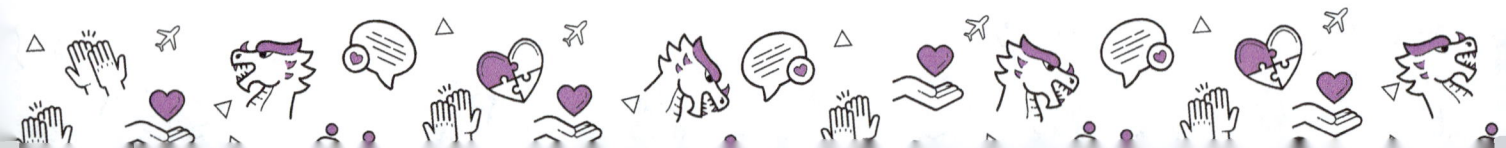

# Social-Emotional Learning Connection

Think about a story, show, movie, song, or social media post you have read or watched over the past 10 weeks that connects to the learning about relationship skills.

What was the source called? _____

How does this text connect to relationship skills and social-emotional learning? Draw a picture or write your answer below.

What was it that made you think about relationship skills? What did you learn about relationship skills from this source?

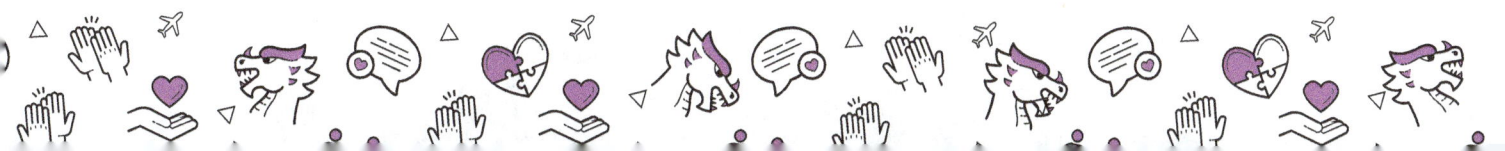

_____

_____

_____

_____

_____

_____

_____

_____

# Notes

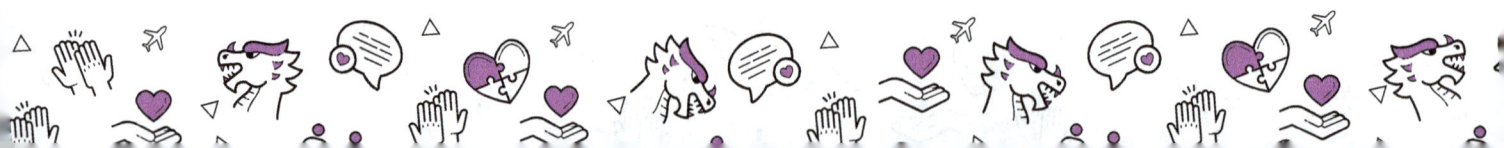

# Notes

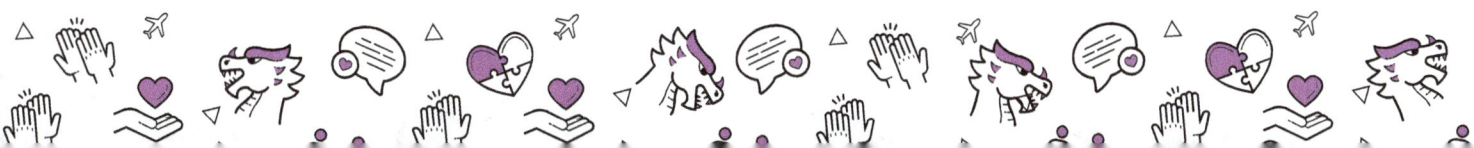

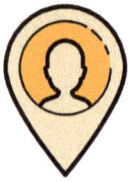

# A Place to Belong

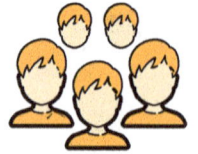

Belonging is a vital element of being human. We all want a place to belong, and as humans, we also have the opportunity to help others feel the sense of belonging. These next 10 weeks, we will focus on the idea of belonging with an emphasis on the social-emotional competency of social-awareness.

**Throughout this theme, you will be exploring:**

1) Appreciating other cultures and perspectives (Appreciating diversity & Perspective-taking)
2) Conflict resolution and communication skills (Empathy & Perspective-taking)
3) Lifting others up and inclusivity (Appreciation diversity, Respect for others, & Perspective-taking)
4) Including everyone (Respect for others & Empathy)
5) Teamwork, collaborating, and maintaining friendships (Perspective-taking & Respect for others)

You belong. The person sitting next to you belongs. We all belong in this world. The theme of belonging is an important one, especially as the world becomes more interconnected. It is important that we all respect each other, include one another when possible, work together, and encourage each other. Here are some ways to explore belonging these next 10 weeks.

**Read:** From your school or community library, check out *Out of my Mind* by Sharon M. Draper. This book is about a girl who has cerebral palsy. This book reminds all of us that everyone deserves to be respected and included. Learn how Melody refuses to be defined by her disability and finds a place to belong in her community.

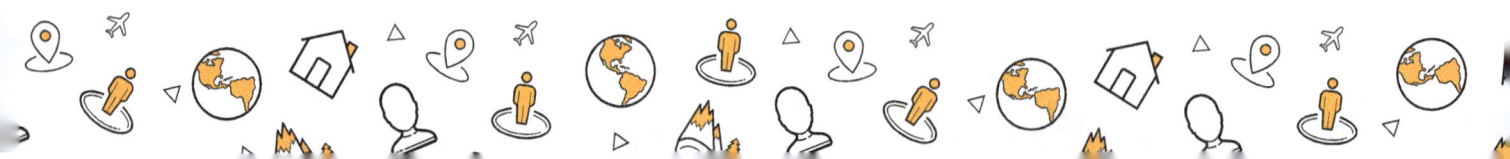

# A Place to Belong

**Listen to:** With your carer's permission, go online to listen to "Ua Roa Te Tau" by Vaiteani. Vaiteani is a Tahitian musical group with upbeat, fun, and relaxing music. If you like the song, you may also be interested in listening to "Horo Horo" and "Belle-Île-en-Mer, Marie-Galante."

How is Vaiteani's music similar to the music you usually listen to? _____

_____

_____

What is your favorite part of this song? _____

_____

_____

How does this song make you feel? _____

_____

_____

**Taste:** People eat different foods all around the world. People usually eat foods that are local to them. Do some research on the types of food a different culture typically eats and then try some new food. Even better: go to a restaurant that serves that culture's food or find a recipe from a cookbook at the library and cook something new with your carer. Appreciate a culture that is not yours with the food you choose to eat.

I tried food from _____

It tasted _____

_____

I would like to try more food from other cultures, including

_____

_____

# Diversity

Diversity is a frequently used word in the media and news. Diversity is the condition of having differing elements, especially the inclusion of different types of people (such as people of different races or cultures) in a group or organization. Many organizations are criticized for not being diverse, not having a variety of genders or ethnicities represented by their members. For example, the Golden Globes, Oscars, and Grammy awards organizations have been widely criticized for the past several years for the lack of nominees from ethnic and gender groups, other than caucasian males.

It is essential to be aware of diversity and the link to what we have learned about relationships, connections, and empathy. No matter what ethnicity you are part of, the acceptance of people who come from different backgrounds is one of the most important lessons, skills, or characteristics we can teach. Think about our discussions about being open to developing friendships and relationships with others. This openness would include everyone you encounter; every ethnicity, age, ability or disability, culture, religion. Everyone, from any type of group, wants to be included, accepted, and connected to others.

**Remember:** One key element in diversity is empathy.

**Activity:** The best way to understand diversity is to understand each other. Use this chart this week to talk to 5 people you don't know and find out more about them. You may find out about yourself and the things you have in common with each other.

| What languages do you speak? | What music do you like to listen to? | What are your favorite foods to eat at home? |
|---|---|---|
| How often do you see your grandparents, cousins, aunts, or uncles? | What holidays do you celebrate in your family? | What values are important to your family? |
| On special occasions or holidays, do you have something special you wear? | What sport or activity does your family enjoy watching or playing? | Are there any games your family plays? |

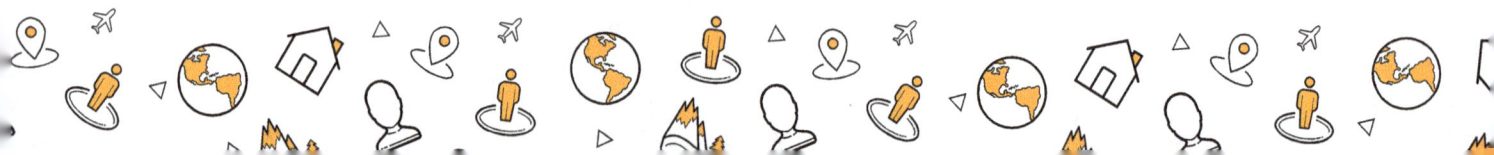

# Homework Log

Week beginning: ___ / ___ / ___

**My goal this week:** _____

_____

| | |
|---|---|
| **Monday** ___ / ___ | |
| **Tuesday** ___ / ___ | |
| **Wednesday** ___ / ___ | |
| **Thursday** ___ / ___ | |
| **Friday** ___ / ___ | |
| **Home/School Communication** | |

# Do You See What I See?

Perspective-taking is a person's ability to consider a situation from a different point of view. It requires you to put yourself in the other person's place in the situation, and imagine what you would feel, think, or do.

Have you ever watched a game on tv, and there was a review of the play to find out what the call should be? The closest referee made the call, but there are cameras all over showing every different view imaginable. The referee could only consider their point of view, and make the call based on what they saw. The people who review the play can look at all the different camera angles and consider every side of the play to decide what the call should be. The result could be to agree with the referee who made the call or to overturn the call that was made based on the different perspectives.

We don't have a review with multiple camera angles to help us understand the point of view of others, but we can practice considering other's points of view before responding. Consider this letter:

# W

What letter do you see? _____ Now turn your paper upside down.
What letter do you see? _____
If you said the letter is W and your friend looked over at your paper and said, "No, that letter is M" what needs to happen, so you both understand each other's perspective?

_____

_____

**Reminder:** Perspective-taking is similar to empathy; you have to consider the other person's thoughts and feelings to understand why they say or do something.

**Activity:** When you were younger, you probably read the classic children's stories like *The Three Pigs, Little Red Riding Hood*, or *The Gingerbread Man*. Take a short story you remember and flip the script. Briefly retell the story from another character's point of view. Some examples of different points of views are below. Share your story with someone.

- The *Gingerbread Man* - Retell the story as the baker
- *Cinderella* - Retell the story as one of the little mice, the prince, or the stepmother
- *Peter Rabbit* - Retell the story from the gardener's point of view

# Homework Log

Week beginning: ___ / ___ / ___

**My goal this week:** _____

_____

| | |
|---|---|
| **Monday** ___ / ___ | _____ _____ _____ _____ |
| **Tuesday** ___ / ___ | _____ _____ _____ _____ |
| **Wednesday** ___ / ___ | _____ _____ _____ _____ |
| **Thursday** ___ / ___ | _____ _____ _____ _____ |
| **Friday** ___ / ___ | _____ _____ _____ _____ |
| **Home/School Communication** | |

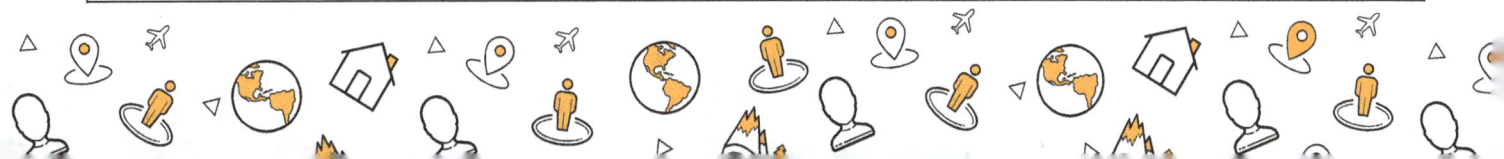

# Conflicts Happen

There are different types of conflict. One type is a conflict we have in our thoughts, feelings, things we want versus things we need is called intrapersonal conflict. The other is interpersonal conflict, which happens when there is a conflict between people. Arguments, disagreements, differences, or fights are all ways we can have interpersonal conflict. Conflict usually happens when two people want different things, or when we feel pulled in our thoughts about two different things we want or need.

**Reminder:** Don't forget about perspective-taking this week. Understanding perspective helps resolve many conflicts. Often, we need to use empathy when others come at us with a conflict.

**Activity:** Think of conflicts you have had, been a part of, or witnessed. Were they intrapersonal (within ourselves) or interpersonal (with others)? Work through these conflicting situations with a classmate, friend, or family member:

At the end of a close game, two basketball players on a team were in a position to score and possibly win the game. One player had the ball, the other player was open to making a shot, but the player with the ball did not throw it to him and took the shot and missed. After the game, they argue about what happened.

Intrapersonal **conflict or** interpersonal **conflict?** _____

**What were the needs in the conflict?** _____

**What were the feelings?** _____

**What was something both sides wanted?** _____

On Friday, you get a text to go to the movies with a friend who had to change schools. You know your mom is working extra hours to pay for something important, and the family budget is tight. You are thinking about the chance to have fun with your friends that you don't get to see very often, and debating how to answer your friend.

Intrapersonal **conflict or** interpersonal **conflict?** _____

**What were the needs in the conflict?** _____

**What were the feelings?** _____

**What was something both sides wanted?** _____

You are walking through the parking lot and find $10.00 lying on the ground. You pick it up and are going to the front desk to turn it in. You meet up with a friend who asks you about the money in your hand. When you tell them you found it, and you are turning it in, they encourage you to keep it or give it to them.

Intrapersonal **conflict or** interpersonal **conflict?** _____

**What were the needs in the conflict?** _____

**What were the feelings?** _____

**What was something both sides wanted?** _____

# Homework Log

Week beginning: ___ / ___ / ___

**My goal this week:** _____

_____

| | |
|---|---|
| **Monday** <br> ___ / ___ | |
| **Tuesday** <br> ___ / ___ | |
| **Wednesday** <br> ___ / ___ | |
| **Thursday** <br> ___ / ___ | |
| **Friday** <br> ___ / ___ | |
| **Home/School Communication** | |

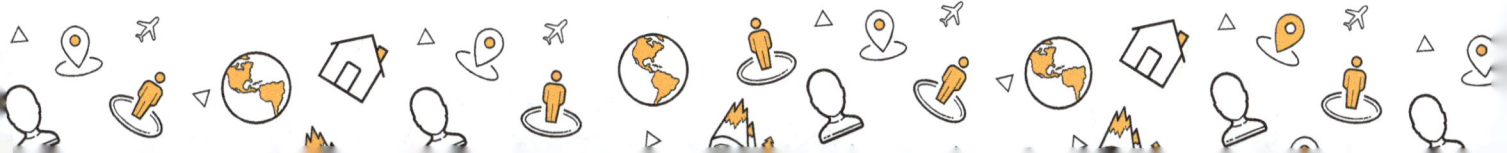

# Can You Hear Me?

Sometimes we experience conflict because we lake critical information about the situation. A key element to understanding and great relationship skills is communication.

One way to listen well to what others are telling us is called reflective listening. To use reflective listening, you give eye contact to the person speaking, give them your attention, nod your head, or use other gestures to show you are engaged in what they are saying. After the person makes a point or a statement, reflect back to them what they have said.

*For example:*

I forgot my homework in math today, and the teacher is making me stay after school today for detention! My mom is going to be so mad because she is going to have to pick me up. What am I going to tell her?

Reflective listening:
Oh, bummer. It sounds like you are having a bad day.

**Reminder:** Don't forget about perspective-taking this week. Understanding perspective helps resolve many conflicts. Often, we need to use empathy when others come at us with a conflict.

**Activity:** Practice reflective listening this week and record instances where you successfully listened with the intent of understanding, not just replying.

I really tried so hard on that test and thought I made a good grade. I spent hours studying and everything. I'm just stupid. I'll never pass this class.

*Reflect:*

So then they said that I took the markers, but I didn't. They just did not believe me. I mean, why would I even want to take the markers? They are always making things up about me to get me into trouble.

*Reflect:*

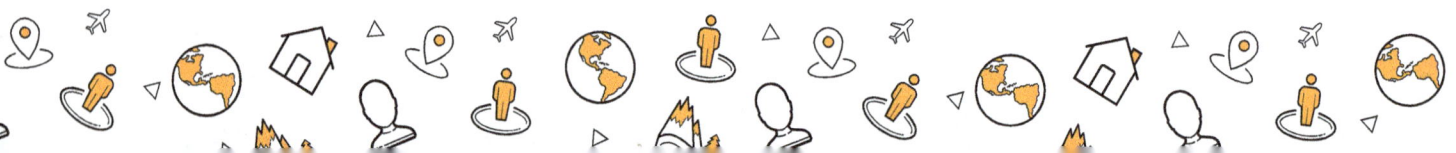

# Homework Log

**My goal this week:** _____

_____

| | |
|---|---|
| **Monday** ___ / ___ | _____<br>_____<br>_____<br>_____ |
| **Tuesday** ___ / ___ | _____<br>_____<br>_____<br>_____ |
| **Wednesday** ___ / ___ | _____<br>_____<br>_____<br>_____ |
| **Thursday** ___ / ___ | _____<br>_____<br>_____<br>_____ |
| **Friday** ___ / ___ | _____<br>_____<br>_____<br>_____ |
| **Home/School Communication** | |

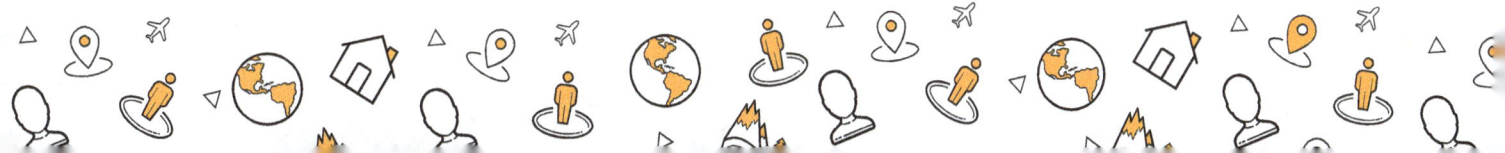

# We Belong

Pause and take a moment to think about a time where you went somewhere new, and you did not know if you would know anyone. You did not know where to sit, who you could talk to, or who would be a friend. Close your eyes and think about how that felt. What feelings did you have?

There is a tendency among people to group up based on sports or activities, culture, and ethnicity, where you live, etc. The list is endless. There is nothing wrong with sharing time with people that share the same interests as you.

Go back to that feeling experience you recalled a few minutes ago. That probably had an uncomfortable feeling, that had a bit of fear, anxiety, anticipation all rolled into one. Was that a good feeling? Would you want that feeling again? Now take that feeling and imagine it happening every day when you are around a group of people that don't include you in their discussion or what they are doing. Can you imagine not feeling welcome?

You can alleviate these negative feelings that others may have simply by showing kindness, and being open to sharing time, even 5 seconds, with others that you may have nothing in common. Once people connect by a smile and a "Hello," it makes room for you to find out what you do have in common. The more you include others, the more you will find that we all belong.

**Activity:** What does belonging mean to you? How can you show acceptance and welcome others to your circle of friends, or your awareness? This week, look for ways to show others they belong by saying hello, asking a sincere question about someone, and showing interest in someone's activities, ideas, or something else about them. What did you find out?

Name of the person: _____

Their response to me saying "Hello": _____

_____

Something they like or enjoy: _____

Something we have in common: _____

How I felt after talking to them: _____

_____

_____

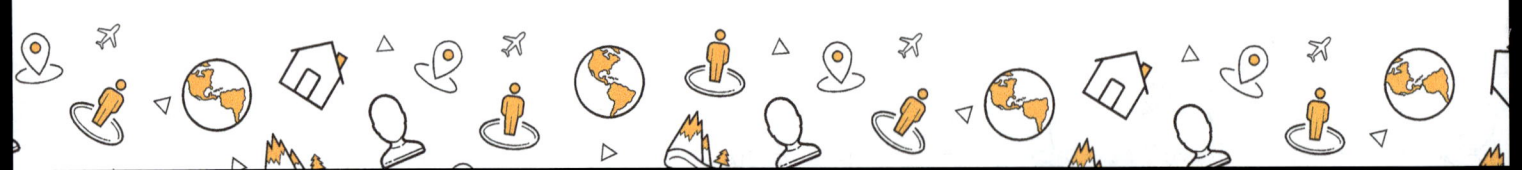

# Homework Log

Week beginning: ___ / ___ / ___

**My goal this week:** _____

_____

| | |
|---|---|
| **Monday**<br>___ / ___ | _____<br>_____<br>_____<br>_____ |
| **Tuesday**<br>___ / ___ | _____<br>_____<br>_____<br>_____ |
| **Wednesday**<br>___ / ___ | _____<br>_____<br>_____<br>_____ |
| **Thursday**<br>___ / ___ | _____<br>_____<br>_____<br>_____ |
| **Friday**<br>___ / ___ | _____<br>_____<br>_____<br>_____ |
| **Home/School Communication** | |

# COLORING

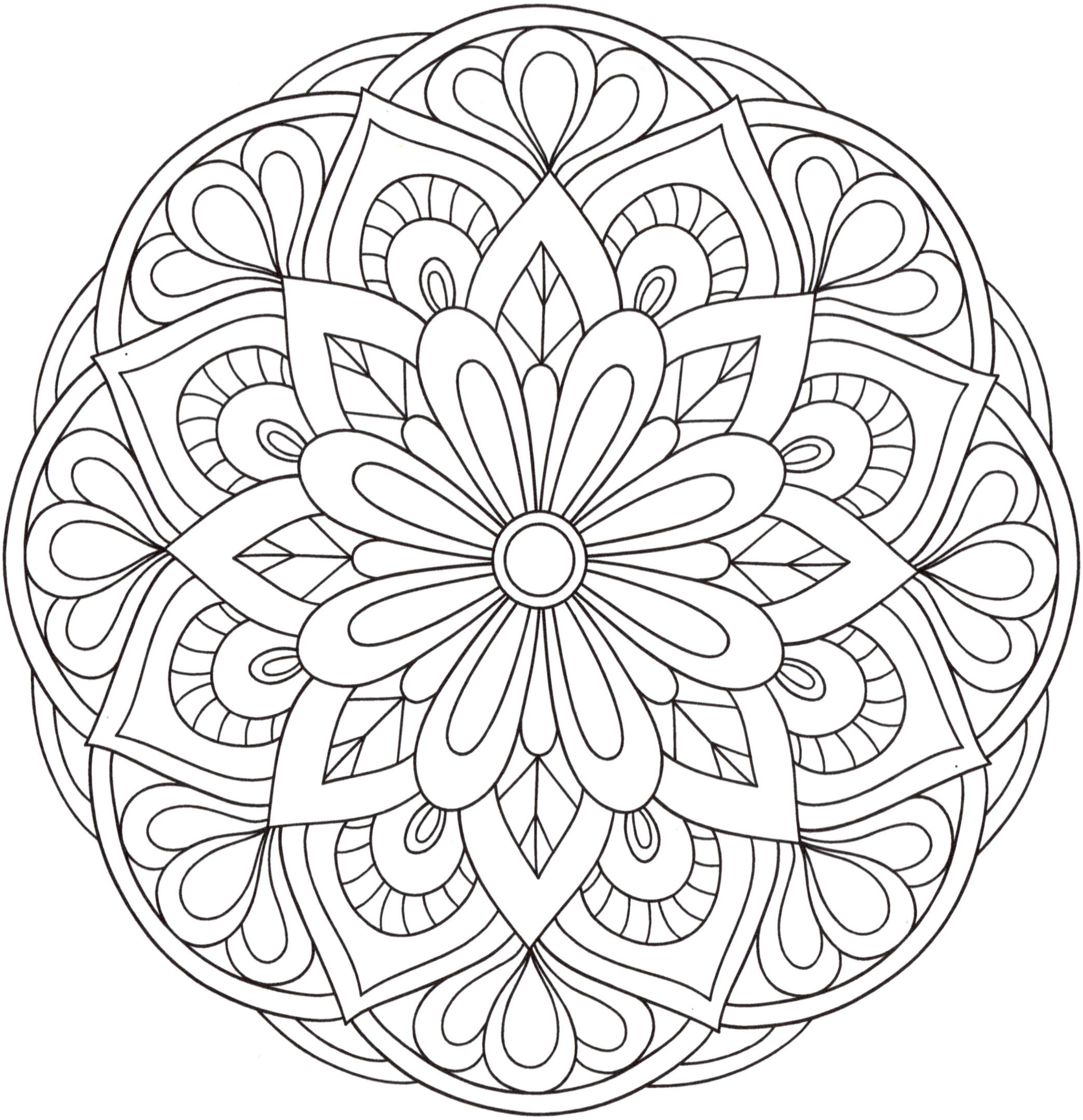

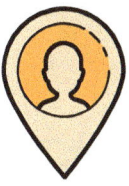

# DOODLING PAGE

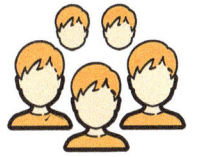

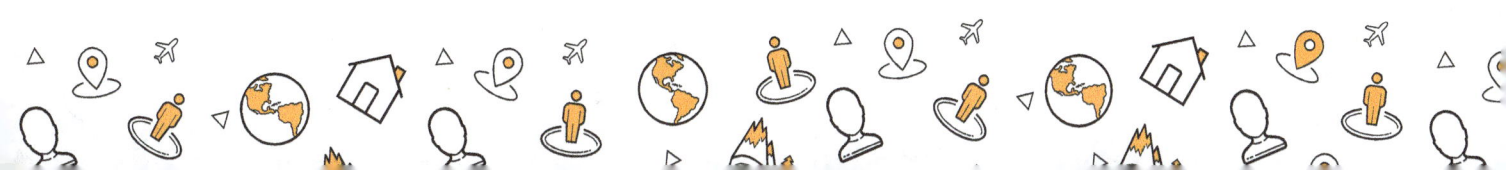

# The Keeping of Friends

One thing middle school students worry about and may experience, is losing a good friend, and we may not even intend to. In middle school, we are separated from our friends by being in different classes, having lockers in different halls, and being involved in different school activities. You can lose touch, grow into different interests, and even make other friends. So, how do we keep a friend?

The key ingredients to keeping a friend are: showing real interest in them and what they do or say, putting them first over others, and continuing to communicate. Showing a real interest in their new activity, or in what they say to you is critical to that person feeling valued by you. Putting the friend first over others means that when you have conflicting plans with a close friend and something another person or event, you try and put your close friend's feelings first.

The need for feeling valued is a key element in keeping a good friend. Show your friends they matter by being interested in them and what they are doing or saying, keep their feelings in mind, and talk to each other to share stories experiences and laughs!

**Activity:** If you have made and lost friends, or have lost touch with a friend, you are not alone. Kids everywhere have the same struggles. Read this question posted by a middle school student. What advice would you give?

Hi, I'm going to middle school this year, and a lot of people tell me you lose and make a lot of new friends. I don't want to lose my best friend. We have been friends for a long time and have been through so much together. I want some tips or advice, please.

_____

_____

_____

_____

_____

_____

_____

_____

_____

# Homework log

Week beginning: ___ / ___ / ___

**My goal this week:** _____

_____

| | |
|---|---|
| **Monday** ___ / ___ | _____<br>_____<br>_____<br>_____ |
| **Tuesday** ___ / ___ | _____<br>_____<br>_____ |
| **Wednesday** ___ / ___ | _____<br>_____<br>_____<br>_____ |
| **Thursday** ___ / ___ | _____<br>_____<br>_____ |
| **Friday** ___ / ___ | _____<br>_____<br>_____<br>_____ |
| **Home/School Communication** | |

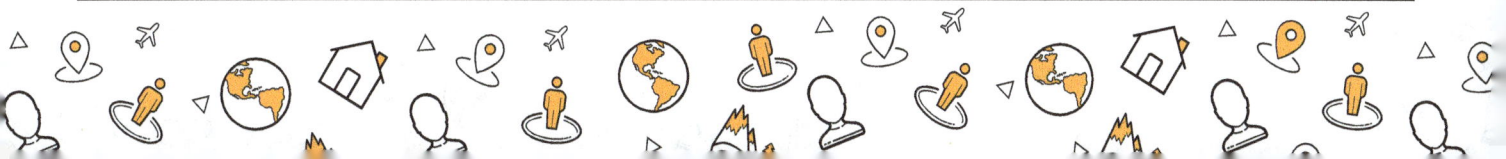

# The Dream Works With Teamwork!

Two words: Group Project. You probably either love group work, or you dread it. People often enjoy group work because they enjoy talking and sharing with others, like to help others, and have others help them. Other people may dread group work for many reasons, one of which is that many times, someone in the group does less work than everyone else! That's not cool. Our focus is on how to work with others successfully without being the person not doing their share. And, to not be the person who does everyone else's work either.

Collaboration means that everyone works together to accomplish a task or a goal. When you work with others and collaborate, you are sharing ideas and listening to a variety of perspectives. You will sometimes be working without a designated leader, and in these groups, you agree on what to do with everyone in the group.

Sometimes people have to be willing to go with someone else's ideas. Teamwork requires trust in the ideas of others and in following through on their part of the work. The team is also going to be trusting in you to do your part, share ideas, and cooperate in finding a solution. You may have to be willing to put your idea aside to go along with someone else's idea.

**Activity:** Play a Game! With your classmates, make two teams. Set up an obstacle course using books and other items between two boundaries, like string. The set up should be a long rectangle shape of obstacles that your teammates will be walking through. One at a time, blindfold a team member and set them at the start of the course. The object is to walk them through the obstacles without stepping out of bounds or on an item. If they do, they have to start over. The team with all players through the course wins!

**Reflect:** How did you work together with your team to place the obstacle game?

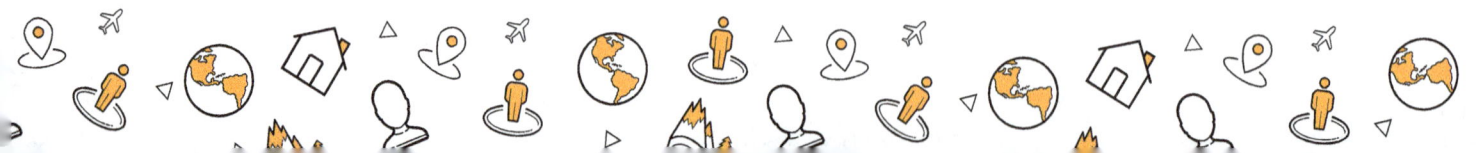

_____

_____

_____

_____

_____

_____

# Homework Log

**My goal this week:** _____

_____

| | |
|---|---|
| **Monday** ___ / ___ | _____ _____ _____ _____ |
| **Tuesday** ___ / ___ | _____ _____ _____ _____ |
| **Wednesday** ___ / ___ | _____ _____ _____ _____ |
| **Thursday** ___ / ___ | _____ _____ _____ _____ |
| **Friday** ___ / ___ | _____ _____ _____ _____ |
| **Home/School Communication** | |

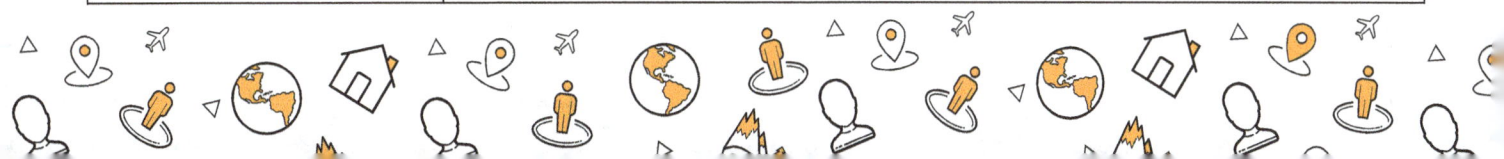

# Let's Hear It For Everyone!

Have you ever watched a football game or a basketball game? When the pressure is on, and the team is down, there are some important people on the sidelines who are yelling louder than before. They are cheering at the top of their voices, standing on each other to be up high so they can be seen and heard better by the team and by the crowd—the cheerleaders. Cheerleaders demonstrate to everyone what needs to be done when teammates, friends, and family get down, have a hard time, and feel like giving up. Cheerleaders show us how important encouragement is to others. They also get other people around them, the fans, to become encouraging. Most of the time, it is the cheerleaders who pump up the crowd, get the band to play an upbeat song, and create a positive atmosphere for the team.

In the locker room, the team has a pep talk before the game and encourages one another to do their best to win. Coaches pump up their players before and during the game. The atmosphere is charged up with good vibes. That atmosphere is carried out of the locker room onto the court or the field with music and cheers.

Encouragement is empathy in action. It's taking how another person feels, and with genuine words of hope, they fill the other person up so they can change how they feel. Encouraging other people around you is a great act of kindness and caring for others. And, you do not even need to know the person you are encouraging!

**Activity:** This week, I challenge you to send a text of encouragement to three people. Say something like, "Hi! I was thinking about you today. I hope you are having a great day!" If you get a reply back, you have to text another person. If you get answers from two people, you have to text two more people, and so on. So for every text you send, you have to send another text to another person. Only count the first reply! If you have restrictions on text messages, use a paper note or a post-it, send a snap or a tweet, etc.

Now, think about the reading above about the team and how they are encouraged by everyone around them. Who do you encourage on the daily?

_____

_____

Who encourages you? _____

_____

If you need someone to cheer you on, let them know!  Sometimes people just do not know what we need, and all we need to do is ask!

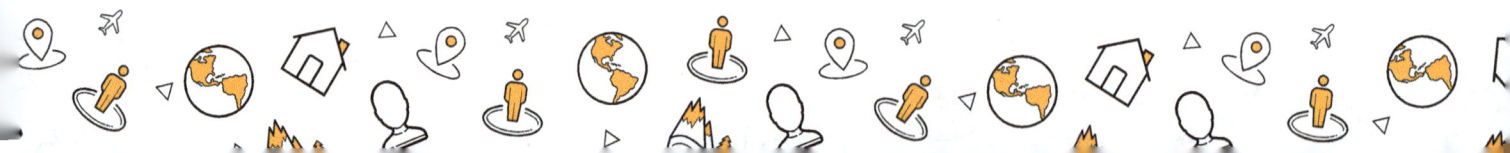

# Homework Log

Week beginning: ___ / ___ / ___

**My goal this week:** _____

_____

| | |
|---|---|
| **Monday** <br> ___ / ___ | |
| **Tuesday** <br> ___ / ___ | |
| **Wednesday** <br> ___ / ___ | |
| **Thursday** <br> ___ / ___ | |
| **Friday** <br> ___ / ___ | |
| **Home/School Communication** | |

# It's Kindness Week!

The focus on kindness this week will hopefully cause waves of kind acts, the "golden rule," that carry on week after week. Have you ever heard of the "golden rule"? It says, in various versions, to treat others as you would have them treat you. It is meant to have us pause and consider how we should treat others, how we should talk to them, what our attitude should be before we act. Another phrase that is often heard is to "put yourself in their shoes," which means to consider the other person first before acting.

There was an experiment at a shopping mall about kindness. Actors had heavy loads to try and carry up a large set of stairs. As they struggled with their bags, a stranger would come by and offer to help them. As they reached the top of the stairs, an amazing thing would happen. Watch and see for yourself in a YouTube video. After getting permission from a parent, teacher, or other caregiver, log in to YouTube and search for "The Everyday Kindness Awards - Stairs".

**Activity:** This week, focus on acts of kindness that are out of ordinary. Challenge yourself and your friends to seek out new ways to be kind. Search for that person at school who seems to be alone and show kindness all week. Here are some suggestions to get you started:

- Bake someone treats.
- Do someone's laundry.
- Make someone a playlist.
- Give someone a book you think they'd like
- Give someone a hug
- Write a list of things you love about someone and give it to them.
- Wash someone's car.

- Babysit, dogsit, or catsit for free.
- Mow someone's lawn.
- Make care packages for the homeless or the military.
- Throw someone a surprise party.
- Bring doughnuts or desserts to school and put them out for others.
- Leave a positive sticky note on someone's desk.

**Reflect:** What acts of kindness did you complete this week? How did you feel after completing each act?

_____

_____

_____

_____

# Homework Log

Week beginning: ____ / ____ / ____

**My goal this week:** _____

_____

| | |
|---|---|
| **Monday** ___ / ___ | _____<br>_____<br>_____<br>_____ |
| **Tuesday** ___ / ___ | _____<br>_____<br>_____<br>_____ |
| **Wednesday** ___ / ___ | _____<br>_____<br>_____<br>_____ |
| **Thursday** ___ / ___ | _____<br>_____<br>_____<br>_____ |
| **Friday** ___ / ___ | _____<br>_____<br>_____<br>_____ |
| **Home/School Communication** | |

# It's Review Week!!

You have covered a lot of important skills to make and maintain healthy relationships. Great work!

What lesson helped you the most?
What information did you read and talk about that you may not have known before?
What activity was the most fun?
What lesson did you apply after that week's lesson was over?

**Activity:** Let's review a few lessons and check how things went.

1) Since learning about being inclusive of others who are different than you in some way, have you learned something you have in common with someone you considered to be different? Have you included any new people into your friendship group?

2) When a difficulty with others happened, did you notice what the needs and feelings were? What were the things both sides wanted, and what happened?

3) Did you try using reflective listening with your friends or family? What happened?

4) How did the kindness challenge go? What kindness activity did you do? Who did you show kindness to? What was their reaction? How did it make you feel?

# Homework Log

Week beginning: ____ / ____ / ____

**My goal this week:** _____

_____

| | |
|---|---|
| **Monday** ___ / ___ | |
| **Tuesday** ___ / ___ | |
| **Wednesday** ___ / ___ | |
| **Thursday** ___ / ___ | |
| **Friday** ___ / ___ | |
| **Home/School Communication** | |

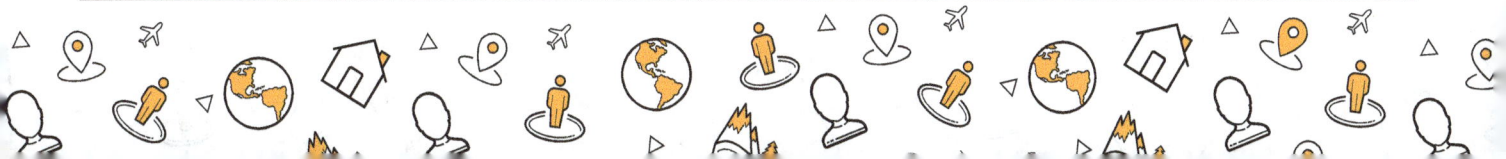

# 10 Week Goal Check-In

Look back at the goals you set for yourself at the beginning of the year or at our last goal check-in. Add notes to check in or make changes to your goals. It's ok to add or change your goals a little, but keep pushing yourself to grow this year. If you feel you have met your goal, make a new goal for yourself at the bottom of this page.

| | How I'm doing on this goal: | What I need to adjust or continue working on: |
|---|---|---|
| Goal: | | |
| Goal: | | |
| Goal: | | |
| Goal: | | |
| Goal: | | |

# Social-Emotional Learning connection

Think about a story, show, movie, song, or social media post you have read or watched over the past 10 weeks that connects to the learning about social-awareness.

What was the source called? _____

How does this text connect to social-awareness and social-emotional learning? Draw a picture or write your answer below.

What was it that made you think about social-awareness? What did you learn about social-awareness from this source?

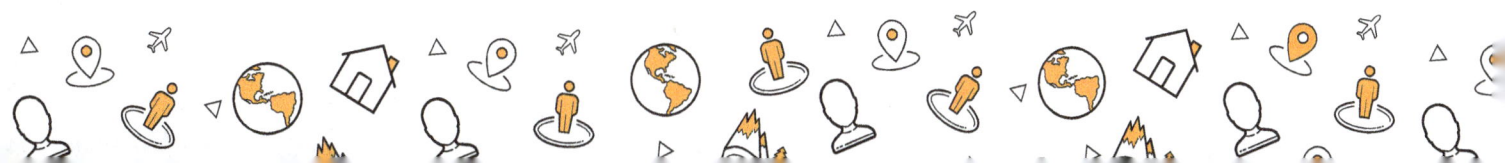

_____

_____

_____

_____

_____

_____

_____

_____

# Notes

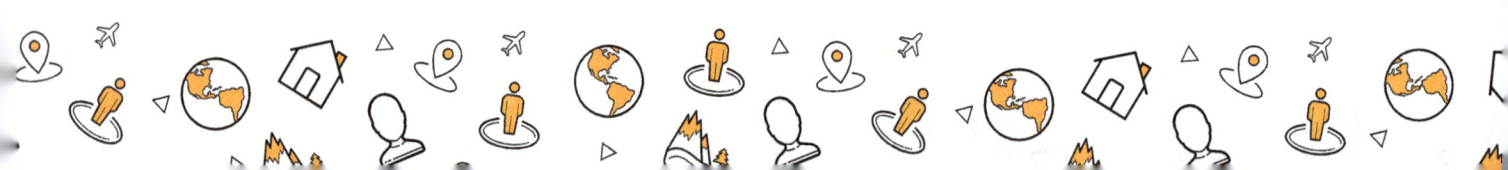

# Notes

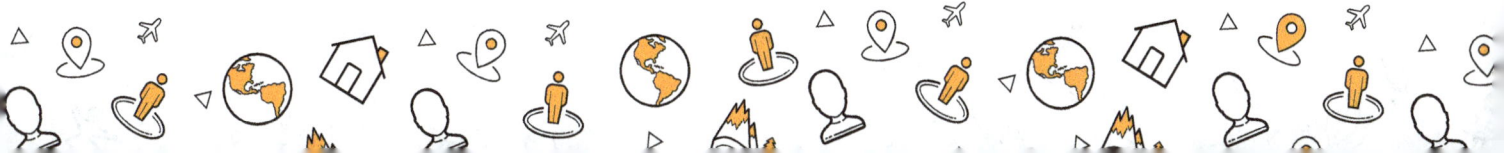

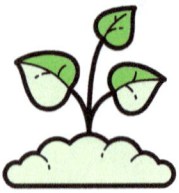
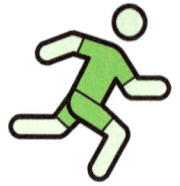

# A Healthy Well-Being

A healthy well-being focuses on all the facets that make you happy. Throughout this theme, the social-emotional competencies emphasized are self-management and responsible decision-making.

Throughout this theme, you will be focusing on:

1) Mindfulness (Impulse control, Stress management, & Self-discipline)
2) Mental health (Identifying problems, Analyzing situations, Solving problems, & Evaluating and reflecting)
3) Coping with stress (Stress management)
4) Passions and strengths (Self-motivation & Evaluating)
5) Perseverance (Solving problems, Self-motivation, & Goal-setting)
6) The place technology and social media has in our lives (Self-discipline, Organizational skills, & Reflecting)
7) Gratitude (Ethical responsibility)

Caring for yourself and ensuring you are healthy on the inside and the outside is important to your overall well-being. Journey through a book, musical piece, and new taste to learn more about well-being.

**Read:** From your school or community library, check out *See you in the Cosmos* by Jack Cheng, a book about a boy's journey to find joy, happiness, and peace within himself. Meet and fall in love with Alex by reading this book to help you understand how well-being doesn't always mean that we will always be happy and get what we want.

**Listen to:** With your carer's permission, go online to listen to "Over the Rainbow" by Hawaiian singer Israel Ka'ano'i Kamakawiwo'ole. This song is a great one to listen to while relaxing, doing some mindfulness, or just slowing down from life.

What did you do while you were listening to this song to help be "well"? _____

_____

_____

What is your favorite part of this song? _____

_____

_____

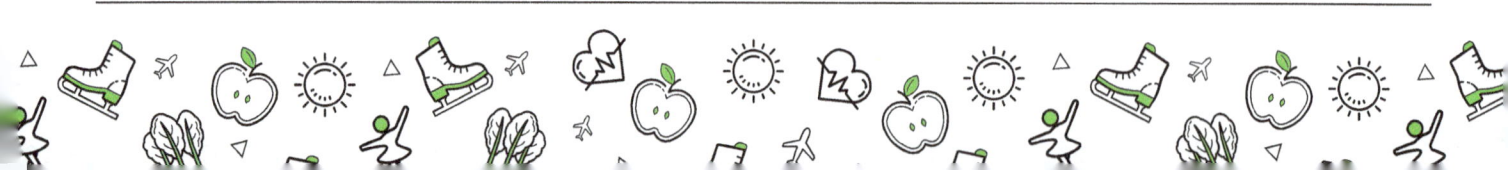

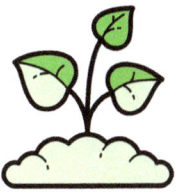

# A Healthy Well-Being

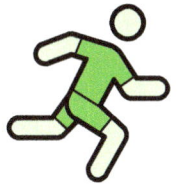

How does this song make you feel? _____

_____

_____

**Taste:** Did you know that about 60% of our bodies are made up of water? Water is important for our bodies to work well. Challenge yourself to drink more water throughout your days. Perhaps you carry a water bottle with you, or you switch from juice to water during meals.

How can you drink more water to be healthier? _____

_____

My goal is to drink _____ ounces of water each day.

After a week or so, reflect on your goal. Are you drinking more water than you did before? _____

_____

## WATER TRACKER

| Day | Amount of Water I Drank | Reflections |
|-----|-------------------------|-------------|
|     |                         |             |
|     |                         |             |
|     |                         |             |
|     |                         |             |
|     |                         |             |
|     |                         |             |

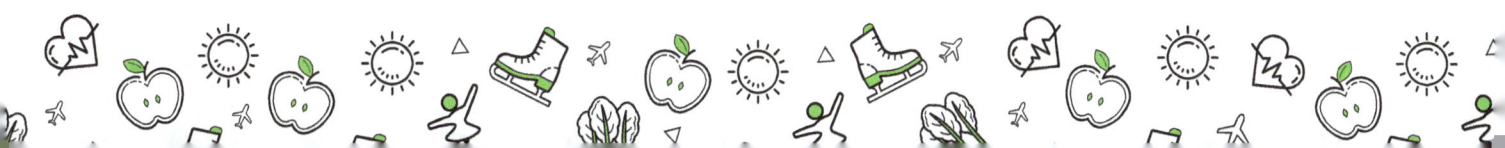

# Where Are Your Thoughts?

When we pay attention to what is going on around us: our thoughts and our physical selves, we are mindful. Mindfulness is a word that you may have heard recently. Mindfulness is paying attention to the present moment: being aware of where we are and what we're doing. Why is this important? When we are mindful, we are less likely to be overwhelmed with things happening around us and distracting thoughts. We can also focus better on what we are doing.

In our world today, people are usually worried about something in the past or the future. You may find yourself upset about a test grade from yesterday, what someone may have said about you or to you, which are "backward" thoughts. You may find yourself feeling anxious about the next test, tryouts, or if someone is your friend, which are "forward" thoughts. When we are thinking backward or forwards, we are not mindful, and we are likely anxious, nervous, upset, or worried. Because we live in a time where we are either thinking "forward" or "backward," we have to spend time practicing thinking about the present and being mindful.

**Activity:** One of the easiest and quickest ways to get to a present state of thinking, or mindfulness, is to focus on your breathing. You can breathe anywhere! There are lots of ways to breathe, and when we concentrate on how we are breathing, we get in tune with where we are, pay attention, and focus. Sit comfortably, close your eyes, and listen to the sound of your breath.

Sit comfortably with one hand over your belly and one hand over your chest. Breathe in slowly and deeply, taking four seconds to breathe in. Hold your breath for seven seconds. Breathe out over eight seconds as quietly as you can and empty your lungs of breath. Repeat at least three times.

Stand up next to your chair or desk. Lean forward and let your arms hang down toward the floor as far as you can. You should be relaxed, not forcing your hands to the floor. Breathe in slowly and slowly stand up, like you are zipping yourself up all the way to the top of your head. Exhale and lean forward with your hands hanging toward the floor again.

How do you feel after these breathing exercises? Do you have a favorite? Try these every day for the week and see how breathing helps you relax and focus.

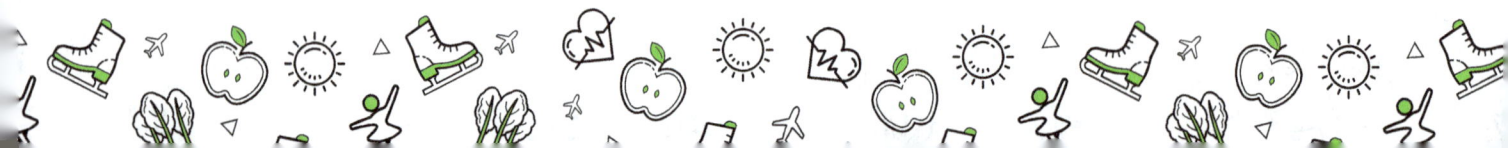

# Homework Log

Week beginning: ___ / ___ / ___

**My goal this week:** _____

_____

| | |
|---|---|
| **Monday** <br> ___ / ___ | _____ <br> _____ <br> _____ |
| **Tuesday** <br> ___ / ___ | _____ <br> _____ <br> _____ |
| **Wednesday** <br> ___ / ___ | _____ <br> _____ <br> _____ |
| **Thursday** <br> ___ / ___ | _____ <br> _____ <br> _____ |
| **Friday** <br> ___ / ___ | _____ <br> _____ <br> _____ |
| **Home/School Communication** | |

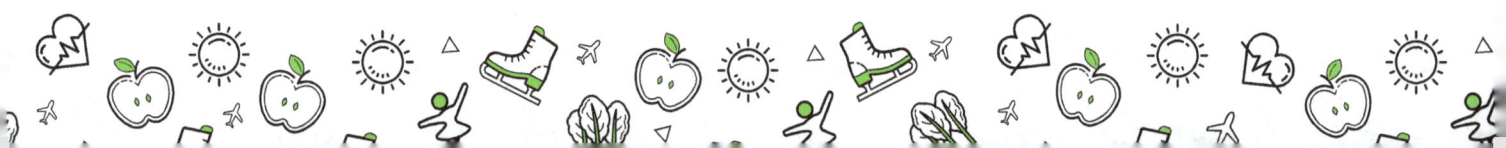

# Your Emotional and Mental Well-Being Are Important

You likely have been sick before with a cold, earache, or stomach ache. When you are sick, you have symptoms. When people have aches and pains, and other symptoms that are from emotional problems, extreme and persistent negative thoughts and feelings, they have a mental illness. Unlike a physical illness, mental illness is not always easy to treat. It can be treated with medicine, and change in thought patterns, but often takes longer to heal than a physical illness.

People can be hurtful, say unkind things, or treat people who have an emotional or mental illness differently. This is called stigmatization. It is one of the top reasons why people who are having emotional problems do not get help. They are afraid of what others will say about them and how they will be treated.

**Activity:** Put a check in the box to mark your opinion. You may be surprised by the answers.

| QUESTION: | STRONGLY DISAGREE | DISAGREE | AGREE | STRONGLY AGREE |
|---|---|---|---|---|
| 1) Anyone can have a mental health problem. | | | | |
| 2) I would be too embarrassed to tell anyone that I had a mental health problem. | | | | |
| 3) People with mental health problems are violent. | | | | |
| 4) If I thought a friend had a mental health problem, I would stay away from them. | | | | |
| 5) I have heard a person I know call someone names like 'nutter,' 'psycho,' 'loony.' | | | | |
| 6) If I thought that I had a mental health problem, I would talk to someone. | | | | |
| 7) Mental health problems only affect adults, not children and young people. | | | | |
| 8) Only certain kinds of people develop mental health problems. | | | | |

1. Anyone can experience a mental health problem. 1/4 people experience one in their life.
2. Embarrassment, and fear of being stigmatized, is a major stumbling block for people who need help with a mental health problem. Yet, being able to talk with someone can help.
3. This is NOT true. This is a pervasive myth. People with mental health problems are much more likely to be victims of violence.
4. Sometimes friends feel that they don't know enough to be able to help or feel uncomfortable. You don't need to be an expert on mental health to be a friend.
5. Such language increases the stigma faced by people experiencing mental health problems and makes it more difficult for them to seek support.
6. A better understanding of mental health problems can reduce the fear, and it is often just very simple, ordinary things that you can do to help a friend.
7. Getting support is a VERY positive factor in treating mental health problems and promoting recovery. It's good to talk!
8. Children and young people may experience mental health problems.

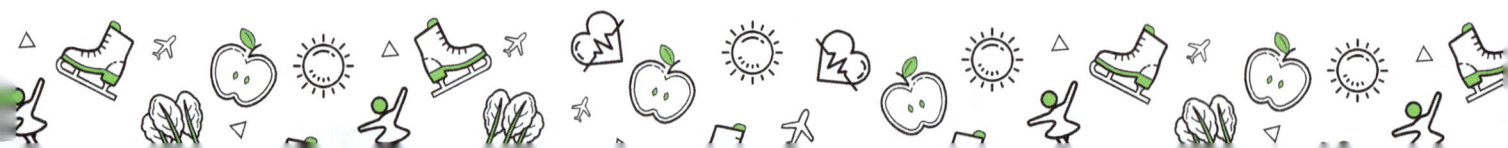

# Homework Log

Week beginning: ____ / ____ / ____

My goal this week: _____

_____

| | |
|---|---|
| **Monday** ___ / ___ | _____<br>_____<br>_____<br>_____ |
| **Tuesday** ___ / ___ | _____<br>_____<br>_____ |
| **Wednesday** ___ / ___ | _____<br>_____<br>_____ |
| **Thursday** ___ / ___ | _____<br>_____<br>_____ |
| **Friday** ___ / ___ | _____<br>_____<br>_____<br>_____ |
| **Home/School Communication** | |

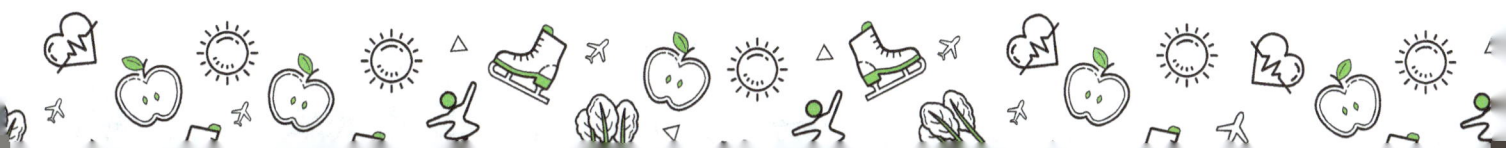

# Find Your Balance

One way to keep ourselves mentally and emotionally healthy is to keep the activities in our lives in balance against each other. Balance in your life is not a 50-50 type of measurement. Sometimes, you may have to stay up late to do your homework, you may stay up late watching a movie with friends, or you may have to stay up for another reason. The balance comes in not staying up that late every night. If you have a baseball bat or a golf club, or a broom, try and balance it on your fingers underneath the object. Your fingers are likely not at the absolute middle of that object, but you have found the spot where that object is in balance. Balance is finding the right amount of what you need to do, required to do, want to do, and rest.

**Activity:** Now that you have made your list, add in the number of hours you spend on each activity. Does your life look balanced? What do you need to do more of? Less of?

| ACTIVITY | HOURS |
|----------|-------|
|          |       |
|          |       |
|          |       |
|          |       |

What areas of your life look balanced? What do you need to do more of? Less of?

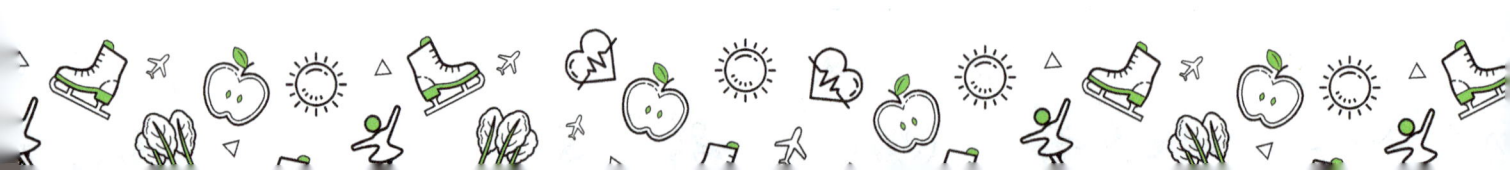

_____

_____

_____

_____

# Homework Log

Week beginning: ___ / ___ / ___

**My goal this week:** _____

_____

| | |
|---|---|
| **Monday**<br>___ / ___ | |
| **Tuesday**<br>___ / ___ | |
| **Wednesday**<br>___ / ___ | |
| **Thursday**<br>___ / ___ | |
| **Friday**<br>___ / ___ | |
| **Home/School Communication** | |

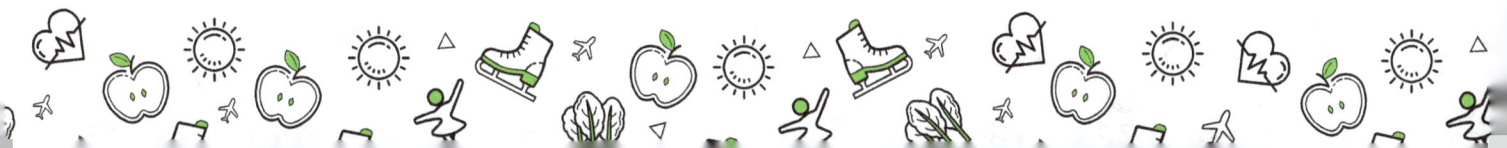

# How Do I Cope?

Our day can be like a maze. We might start well, maybe we made our bed, ate a good breakfast, and had our homework ready, but then… smack! We hit a barrier. Perhaps there is a pop quiz, there is a substitute teacher that may sound unfriendly, or we don't like what is served for lunch. So, what do you do?

You have a choice - you can either Cope or Cop-out. Coping is dealing with unexpected things that may stop us from doing something we expected to do. Copping-out is when you choose to avoid the problem, make excuses, or put up a barrier of your own by yelling, using harsh words, or having a bad attitude. Coping will help us deal with unexpected situations; copping-out will add to our difficulties. Each time we choose how we deal with barriers is like a maze; we can go one way and cope, or another way and cop-out. One way will lead to good decisions and keep us moving, and the other way will lead us to more barriers.

**Activity:** Think about yesterday, last week, or any time where you can reflect on how you responded to unexpected situations. What did you do? How did you respond? Did you cope or cop-out? How did that work out? Remember, just because we cope with a barrier does not mean it removes the problem, it means we can keep going.

| BARRIER | COPE OR COP-OUT? | WHAT HAPPENED NEXT? | DID IT HELP OR HURT? |
|---------|------------------|---------------------|----------------------|
|         |                  |                     |                      |
|         |                  |                     |                      |
|         |                  |                     |                      |

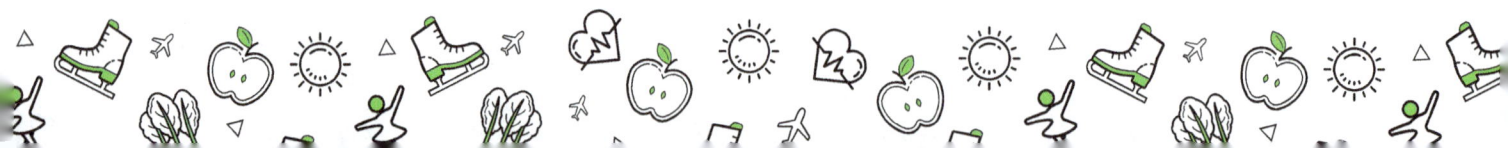

# Homework Log

Week beginning: ____ / ____ / ____

My goal this week: _____

_____

| | |
|---|---|
| **Monday** ___ / ___ | _____<br>_____<br>_____<br>_____ |
| **Tuesday** ___ / ___ | _____<br>_____<br>_____ |
| **Wednesday** ___ / ___ | _____<br>_____<br>_____ |
| **Thursday** ___ / ___ | _____<br>_____<br>_____ |
| **Friday** ___ / ___ | _____<br>_____<br>_____ |
| **Home/School Communication** | |

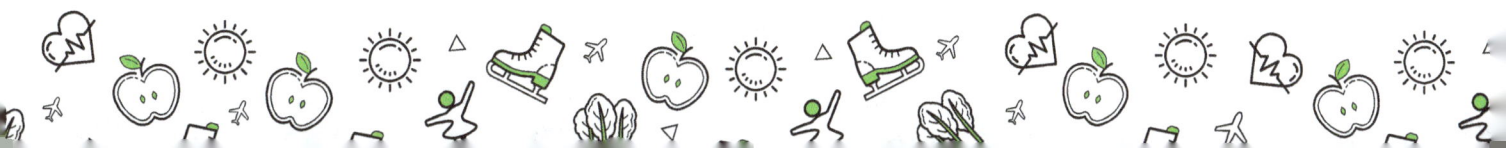

# Strengths and Passions

To have strength is to have a quality of being able to do hard things. These things can be physical, mental, or emotional. Strength is also about having the energy and determination to meet a challenge. A strength does not have to be off the charts awesome. It can be an area of your abilities that is better than your other skills and abilities. Sometimes our strengths are not flashy, like lifting heavyweights. Strengths can be of your character, such as patience, responsibility, and caring. Passions are activities you enjoy so much that setting your alarm and waking up to go out and engage in the activity is not a problem that you love to do.

Your strengths and passions bring us back to the topic of identity. Things we love to do, and things we are good at, describe us and sometimes define us. If you are really great at math, in group projects, you may be the "math person." If you are super at tumbling and gymnastics, you may be referred to someone you meet for the first time as "the gymnast." We can start to think about the future by focusing on these skills and interests and trying to integrate them into an activity or job we would be great at and enjoy.

**Activity:** In the Venn Diagram below, add your Strengths in the left circle and your Passions in the right circle. Then note how these strengths & passions relate to each other. For example, if I love jumping and doing flips, and I am physically strong, these can go together if I were a gymnast.

Where the two circles intersect above, write possible activites or professions that relate to both your strengths & passions.

# Homework Log

Week beginning: ___ / ___ / ___

My goal this week: _____

_____

| | |
|---|---|
| **Monday** ___ / ___ | |
| **Tuesday** ___ / ___ | |
| **Wednesday** ___ / ___ | |
| **Thursday** ___ / ___ | |
| **Friday** ___ / ___ | |
| **Home/School Communication** | |

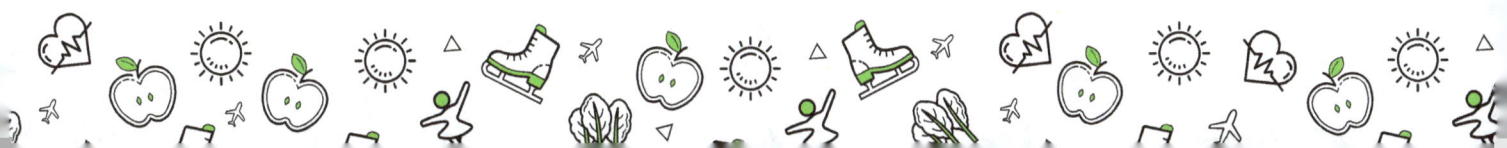

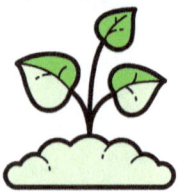

# COLORING

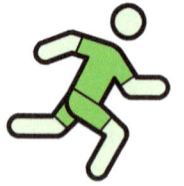

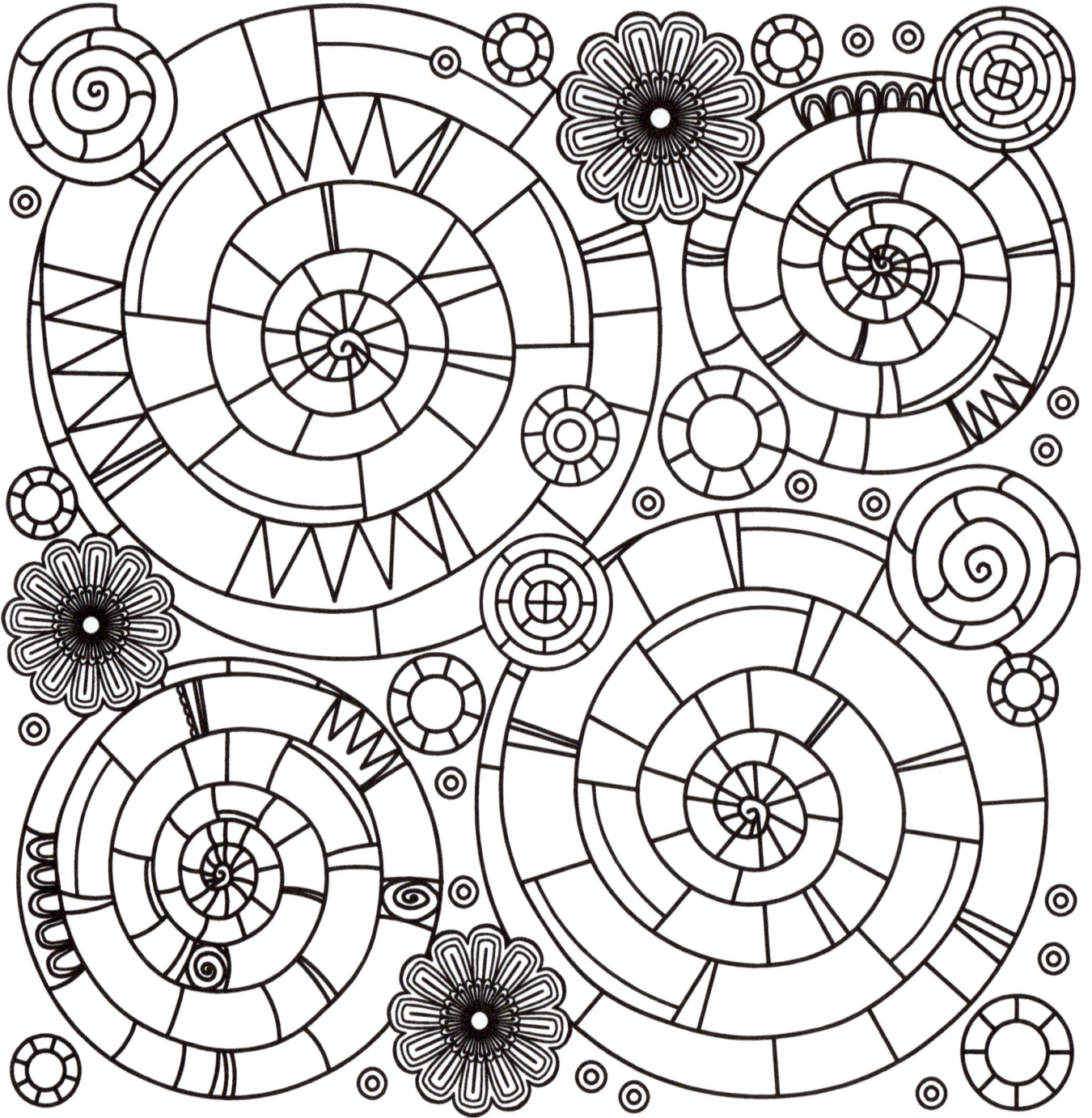

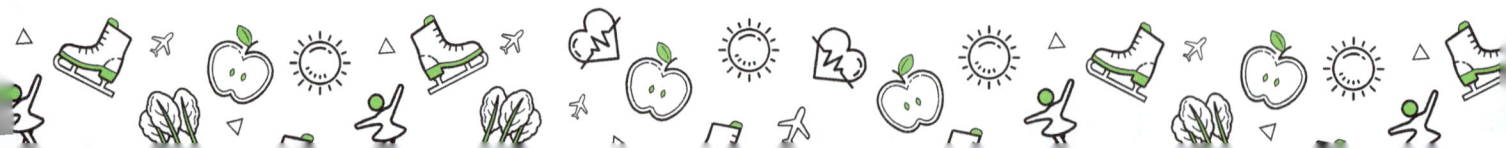

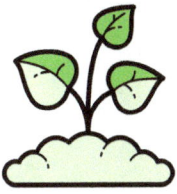

# DOODLING PAGE

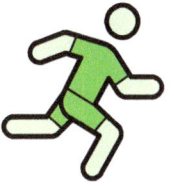

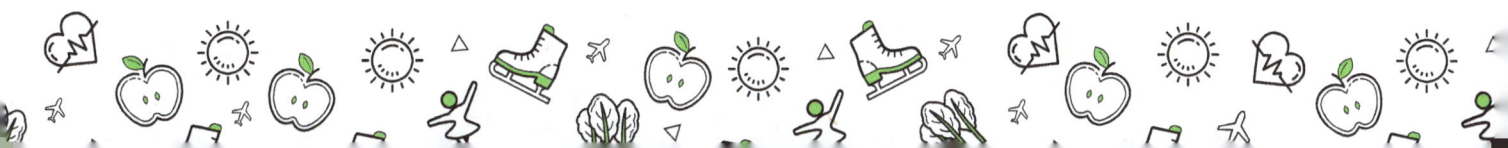

# Decisions, Decisions!

How many decisions did you make today? You will likely make more than 3,000 decisions in one day! Research says you will make about 200 decisions alone about what food to eat daily. How do we make so many choices in a short amount of time?

Much of the time, we make decisions out of habit, something we have always done. We might make impulsive choices without thinking. We might decide NOT to make a decision, or we might let someone else decide for us. These are the easy choices that go by us so fast; we might not even notice. The best decisions are made when we consider what is best for us at the time, what is best for other people and how it will affect them, or when we consider how the decision will affect our future. These are considered responsible decisions.

**Activity:** For decisions that need some thought, what is your decision-making style? How do you approach decisions regularly? Do you change styles depending on what the choice is? Or do you avoid decisions and choose NOT to decide?

| DECISION-MAKING STYLE: | DECISIONS I MAKE WITH THIS STYLE: |
|---|---|
| **REACTIONARY** - I ask others what they would do and do what they suggest. | |
| **IMPULSIVE** - I don't really think about it. I just do whatever comes to mind. | |
| **FATALISTIC** - I just wait and see what happens. I don't think my decision will change anything. | |
| **PROCRASTINATE** - I wait until the last minute before making a decision, and I usually change my mind several times. | |
| **PLANNING** - I take a lot of time to decide and work through every possible solution or action. | |
| **INTUITIVE** - You let your feelings decide. Your decisions may be made by intuition or how you feel about the decision. | |

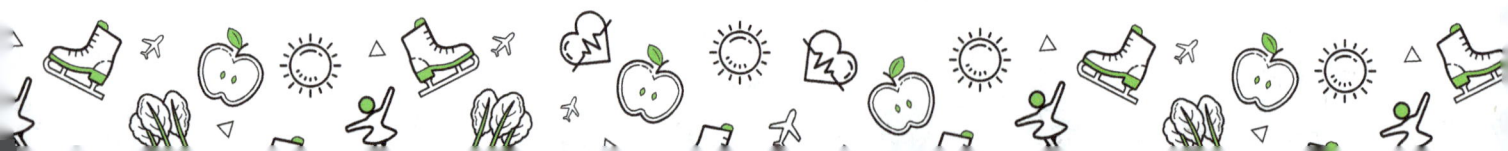

# Homework Log

Week beginning: ____ / ____ / ____

My goal this week: _____

_____

| | |
|---|---|
| **Monday** ___ / ___ | _____<br>_____<br>_____<br>_____ |
| **Tuesday** ___ / ___ | _____<br>_____<br>_____<br>_____ |
| **Wednesday** ___ / ___ | _____<br>_____<br>_____<br>_____ |
| **Thursday** ___ / ___ | _____<br>_____<br>_____<br>_____ |
| **Friday** ___ / ___ | _____<br>_____<br>_____<br>_____ |
| **Home/School Communication** | |

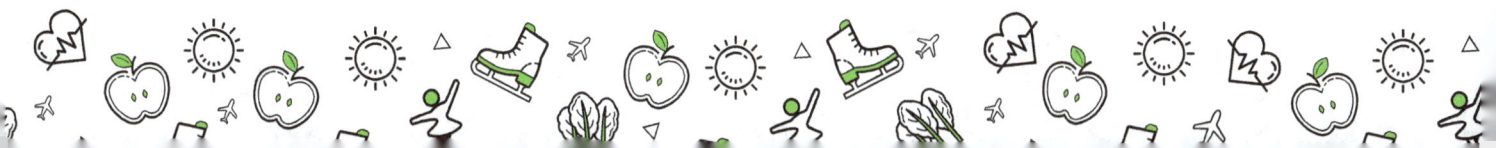

# I Dare You

The Pew Research Center has reported that 45% of teens say they're online almost constantly. We know that technology is being used more than ever, more often than ever. You may use your phone or a device in class today. Many people have stopped using a home phone and only have their cell phones.

The thing is, as technology use increases, something else must be decreasing. For example, if we spend four hours between our cell phone, watching shows on tv, and searching for things online, that is four hours we were not interacting in a meaningful way with others. That's four hours we may not have connected personally with our family.

Many middle schoolers are spending 89% of the day on the phone. During the hours you are awake, you are at school approximately 8 hours, on the bus or traveling to school for approximately 1.5 hours, eating for about 1.5 hours, and engaged in other activities for about 5 hours of the day, besides sleeping. The total time of your day awake and active is approximately 16 hours; 89% of 16 hours is 14 hours and 24 minutes that you are on your phone or another technology device!

---

**Activity:** Make a realistic plan for taking a break from technology.

---

To limit my screen time, I will _____

_____

With the "extra" time you have by not being on your phone, build your skills in intentionally taking time for you and others without distractions.

**In the cafeteria, I can...**
- Help someone with their homework.
- 
- 
- 

**In the car, I can...**
- Take turns choosing the music.
- 
- 
- 

**Before bed, I can...**
- Pack my backpack for tomorrow.
- 
- 
- 

**At dinner with my family, I can...**
- Share the highlights of my day.
- 
- 
-

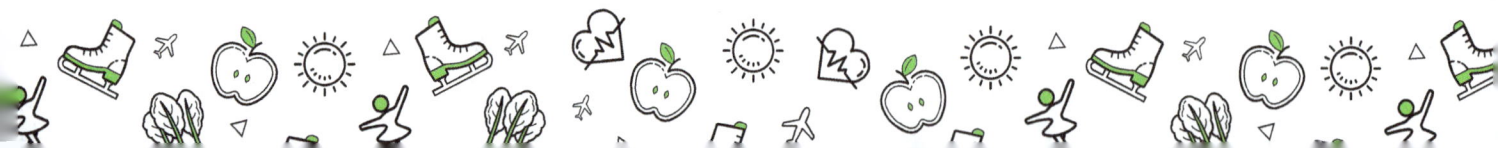

# Homework Log

Week beginning: ___ / ___ / ___

My goal this week: _____

_____

| | |
|---|---|
| **Monday** <br> ___ / ___ | _____ <br> _____ <br> _____ <br> _____ |
| **Tuesday** <br> ___ / ___ | _____ <br> _____ <br> _____ <br> _____ |
| **Wednesday** <br> ___ / ___ | _____ <br> _____ <br> _____ <br> _____ |
| **Thursday** <br> ___ / ___ | _____ <br> _____ <br> _____ <br> _____ |
| **Friday** <br> ___ / ___ | _____ <br> _____ <br> _____ <br> _____ |
| **Home/School Communication** | |

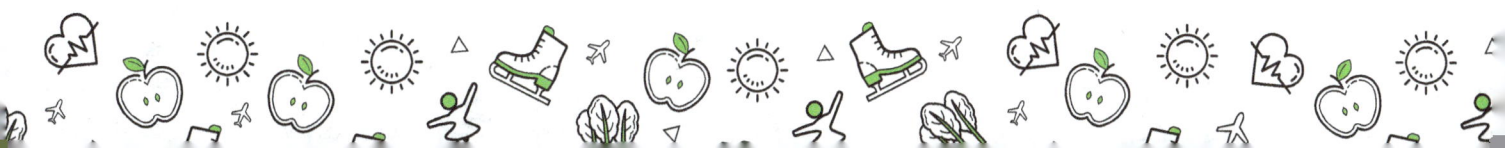

# Cyber Safety on Social Media

There are things that students need to be aware of when they interact on any form of social media to stay safe. Safe from what? (Glad you asked!) To stay safe from identity theft and people who look on all social media platforms to find students like you for bad intentions. People in your life value you and your safety is a concern.

There are several ways to protect yourself on social media by NOT posting:

▸ Your full birthday with the year given. Use a fake birthdate or at least a fake year.
▸ Relationship status. I know, are people really in a relationship if they do not post it on social media? If you must post it, don't use the last name or tagging.
▸ Address. Never give your address and personal information to anyone. That means people on social media.
▸ Phone number. Send your phone number via message or text it to them.
▸ Where you are. Turn off the map location on apps. This is certainly the first way someone would be able to find you.
▸ Where and when you are going on vacation. Don't let people know when it will be easy for them to rob your home!

**Activity:** Get your safety check done!

First, take this online quiz to see how you do: http://www.safekids.com/quiz/.

Now, check your safety. Different versions and brands of phones have security functions built-in them. It would be great to talk to the store where your phone came from and ask the professional about running a safety check. Update your passwords often and do not reply to unusual messages. Go through these and other safety instructions from other apps you may have that are not on this list. Use these sites to learn how to secure your apps.

**Snapchat:** https://www.snap.com/en-US/safety/safety-center/.

**Tik Tok:** https://www.internetmatters.org/parental-controls/social-media/tiktok-privacy-and-safety-settings/.

**Instagram:** https://about.instagram.com/community/safety.

**Facebook**: https://www.facebook.com/help/122006714548814?helpref=popular_topics.

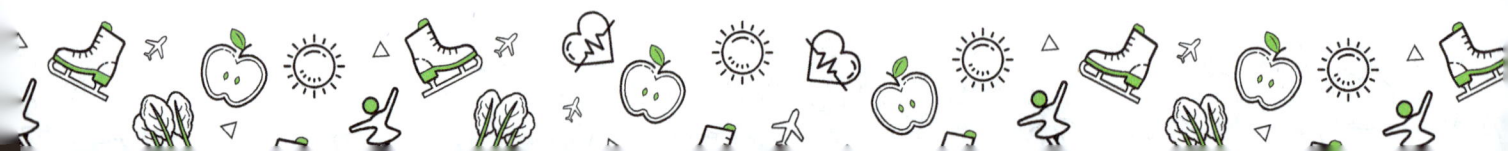

# Homework Log

Week beginning: ___ / ___ / ___

**My goal this week:** _____

_____

| | |
|---|---|
| **Monday** ___ / ___ | _____<br>_____<br>_____<br>_____ |
| **Tuesday** ___ / ___ | _____<br>_____<br>_____<br>_____ |
| **Wednesday** ___ / ___ | _____<br>_____<br>_____<br>_____ |
| **Thursday** ___ / ___ | _____<br>_____<br>_____<br>_____ |
| **Friday** ___ / ___ | _____<br>_____<br>_____<br>_____ |
| **Home/School Communication** | |

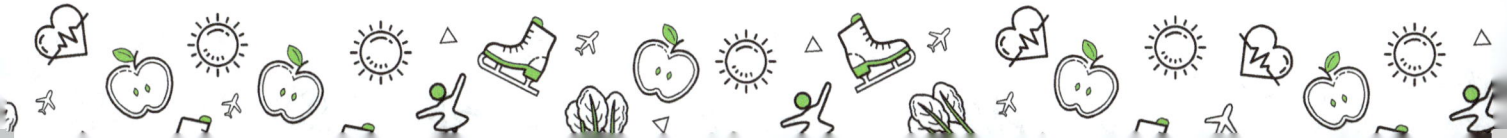

# Gratitude is a Heart Attitude

Being grateful is a feeling of thankfulness that we experience when we appreciate a person or a thing. Often we feel gratitude when we receive something, like a gift. Gratitude can also be a way of being. You can have an attitude of gratitude regularly, for people in your life, for things you have, opportunities that you can enjoy, for your strengths and passions, for your friends and family. The list is literally endless.

Gratitude is important, not just to show thankfulness for receiving something, but it benefits our mental and emotional wellbeing. A lot of research has been done on how being grateful helps us.

▸ People who exhibit gratitude take better care of their own health and feel healthier
▸ Gratitude creates an opportunity to meet more people and form connections
▸ Toxic emotions decrease in our mind, and we have more feelings of happiness
▸ People sleep better and longer
▸ Gratitude helps improve self-esteem by reducing how we compare ourselves to others and increase our ability to accept and be grateful for our own skills
▸ Gratitude improves our mental strength and determination by helping people overcome stress and trauma
▸ Our ability to empathize with other people increases and people act with more kindness

**Activity:** Every day this week, write a note of gratitude and thanks to someone at school and home. Think past the obvious people like your close friends. Write a note and post it on lockers of someone new to your school, the campus maintenance staff and cafeteria workers who work hard behind the scenes of the campus; the office staff and school nurse who have to take care of many problems every day and keep the school running.

Everyday this week, write in your planner three things you are grateful for. Try and make this a habit of continuing it every day.You can write in this planner on the following page titled Gratitude Journal. Try and always think of three things.

**Reflect:** How do you feel at the end of the week? Did anyone notice the notes you left? How did it feel to write to them? Did you write three things you were thankful for in your planner? Continue this practice of gratitude and notice what difference you observe after a few more weeks.

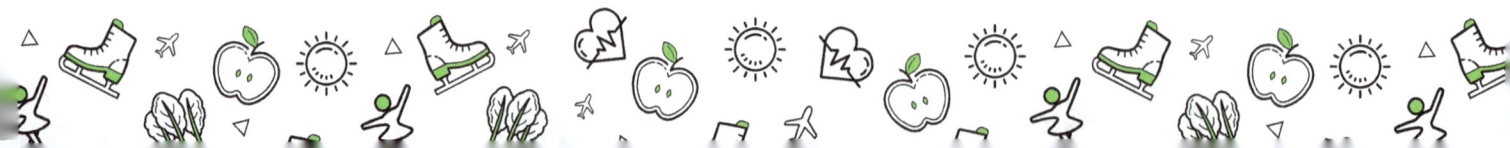

_____

_____

_____

_____

# Homework Log

Week beginning: ____ / ____ / ____

**My goal this week:** _____

_____

| | |
|---|---|
| **Monday** ___ / ___ | |
| **Tuesday** ___ / ___ | |
| **Wednesday** ___ / ___ | |
| **Thursday** ___ / ___ | |
| **Friday** ___ / ___ | |
| **Home/School Communication** | |

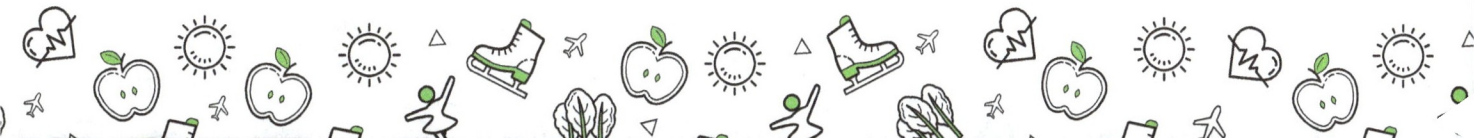

# Gratitude Journal

Gratitude is the practice of being thankful. It's most powerful when it's shared. When practiced daily, it can lead to more happiness. Use these two pages to begin your gratitude journal.

_____

_____

_____

_____

_____

_____

_____

_____

_____

_____

_____

_____

_____

_____

_____

_____

_____

_____

_____

_____

_____

_____

_____

_____

# Gratitude Journal

# Our Last Review Week!

This week is bitter-sweet as we look back on our learning. You did great work by trying to apply things that may have seemed unusual and to take care of your personal safety.

1) If you had to title your last 9 weeks of Social-Emotional Learning, what title would you give your learning?

   _____

2) What lesson was challenging this 9 weeks? What made it a challenge?

   _____

3) Were you inspired to do more, try something new, or make a change in your daily life this 9-weeks? What was it? What did you do?

   _____

4) Looking at your balance from a few weeks ago, and thinking about it now, were you able to do something to get more balance? What area? How did you accomplish that?

   _____

5) When reducing your time with technology, how much time did you increase to spend with family and friends, or in doing other activities? How did that feel?

   _____

**Activity:** What did you learn about yourself over the past school year? Describe what you learned about your body, mind, emotions, relationships, academics, and attitude.

| _My Body_ | _My Mind_ |
|---|---|
| _My Emotions_ | _My Relationships_ |
| _My Academic Success_ | _My Attitude_ |

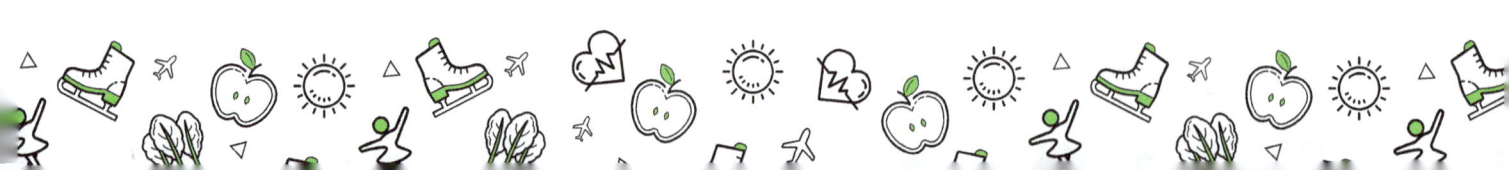

# Homework Log

Week beginning: ____ / ____ / ____

**My goal this week:** _____

_____

| | |
|---|---|
| **Monday** ___ / ___ | _____<br>_____<br>_____<br>_____ |
| **Tuesday** ___ / ___ | _____<br>_____<br>_____<br>_____ |
| **Wednesday** ___ / ___ | _____<br>_____<br>_____<br>_____ |
| **Thursday** ___ / ___ | _____<br>_____<br>_____<br>_____ |
| **Friday** ___ / ___ | _____<br>_____<br>_____<br>_____ |
| **Home/School Communication** | |

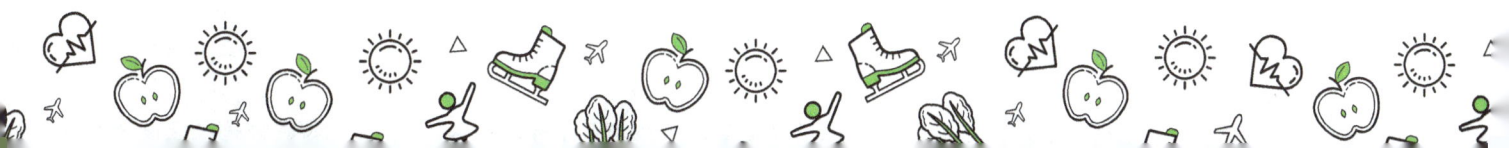

# 10 Week Goal Check-In

Look back at the goals you set for yourself at the beginning of the year or at our last goal check-in. Add notes to check in or make changes to your goals. It's ok to add or change your goals a little, but keep pushing yourself to grow this year. If you feel you have met your goal, make a new goal for yourself at the bottom of this page.

| | How I'm doing on this goal: | What I need to adjust or continue working on: |
|---|---|---|
| Goal: | | |
| Goal: | | |
| Goal: | | |
| Goal: | | |
| Goal: | | |

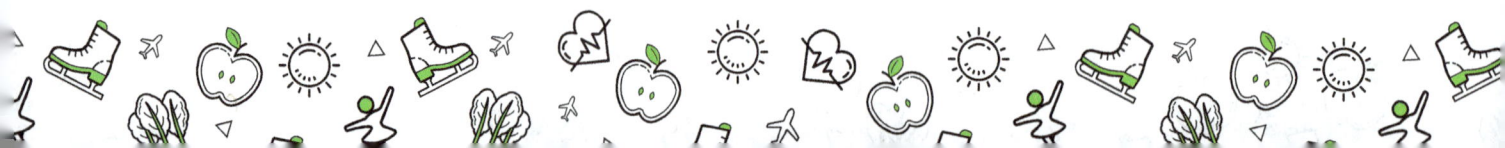

# Social-Emotional Learning Connection

Think about a story, show, movie, song, or social media post you have read or watched over the past 10 weeks that connects to the learning about self-management or responsible decision-making.

What was the source called? _____

How does this text connect to self-management or responsible decision-making and social-emotional learning? Draw a picture or write your answer below.

What was it that made you think about self-management or responsible decision-making? What did you learn about it from this source?

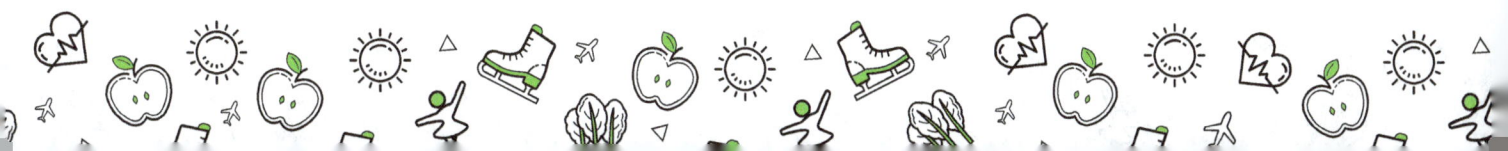

_____

_____

_____

_____

_____

_____

_____

_____

# Notes

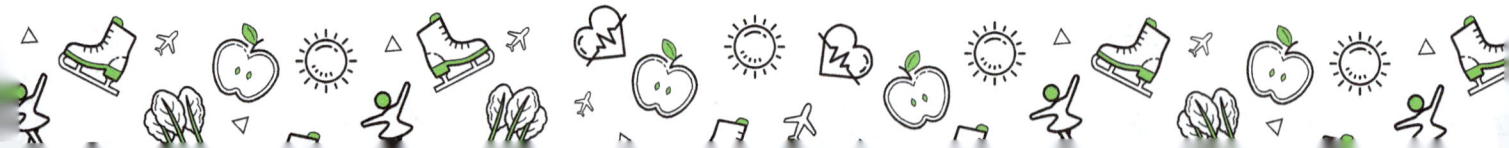

# Notes

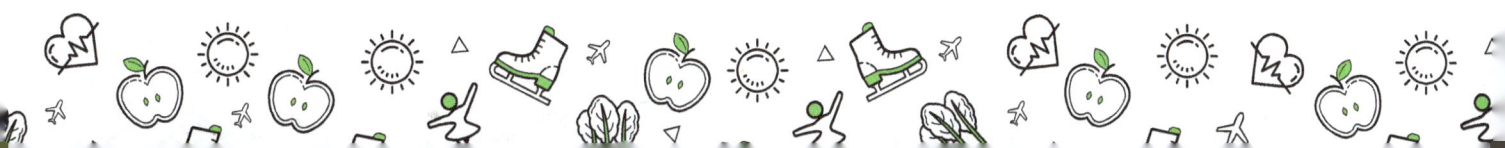

# A Look Back on 7th Grade

Hooray! You completed 7th grade! CONGRATULATIONS!! How do you feel? Did this school year feel like it went by fast or slow? 7th grade was full of events that made an impact on you. As this year ends, take some time to think about these questions and talk about them with a friend, your class, or your family.

1) What were the top three things that happened this school year?

_____

_____

2) What were some of the hardest parts of your school year?

_____

_____

3) Who was part of your support system; people who you counted on for help?

_____

_____

4) What is something you remember most from your social and emotional lessons? What is the most important thing you learned?

_____

_____

5) What would you tell the students in 6th grade about 7th grade?

_____

_____

6) Next year, you will be in 8th grade, which is a special year. What are you most looking forward to?

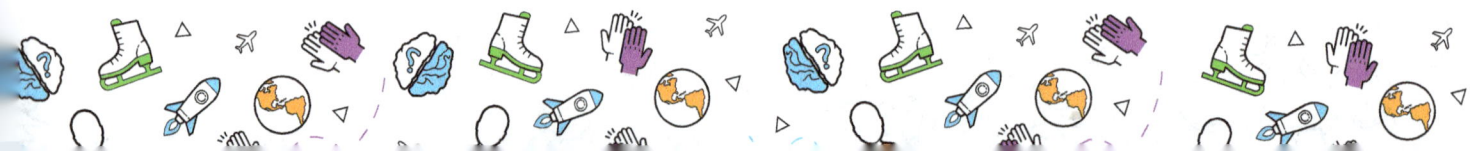

_____

_____

# A Look Back on 7th Grade

**Goal #1:** _____

Reflection on my goal: _____

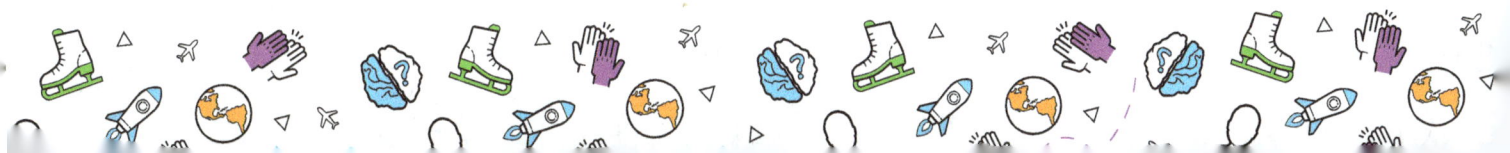

_____

_____

_____

**Goal #2:** _____

Reflection on my goal: _____

_____

_____

_____

**Goal #3:** _____

Reflection on my goal: _____

_____

_____

_____

# Activity Tracker

Use this activity tracker to record the sports, clubs, and other programs you are involved in this year. Remembering your activities is helpful when you apply for a special program, activity or opportunity.

| DATE STARTED | DATE ENDED | ACTIVITY | HOURS | DESCRIPTION/TEACHER OR COACH SIGNATURE |
|---|---|---|---|---|
| | | | | |
| | | | | |
| | | | | |
| | | | | |
| | | | | |
| | | | | |
| | | | | |
| | | | | |
| | | | | |
| | | | | |
| | | | | |
| | | | | |
| | | | | |
| | | | | |
| | | | | |
| | | | | |
| | | | | |
| | | | | |

# Service Learning

Track all your service learning throughout the year. Use the description area to give more details about what you did or what organization you worked with so you can remember in the future. If you need a signature to verify your hours, you can use the description area for the service learning coordinator to sign off your hours.

| DATE | SERVICE LEARNING ACTIVITY | HOURS | DESCRIPTION/SUPERVISOR'S SIGNATURE |
|------|---------------------------|-------|-----------------------------------|
|      |                           |       |                                   |
|      |                           |       |                                   |
|      |                           |       |                                   |
|      |                           |       |                                   |
|      |                           |       |                                   |
|      |                           |       |                                   |
|      |                           |       |                                   |
|      |                           |       |                                   |
|      |                           |       |                                   |
|      |                           |       |                                   |
|      |                           |       |                                   |
|      |                           |       |                                   |
|      |                           |       |                                   |
|      |                           |       |                                   |
|      |                           |       |                                   |
|      |                           |       |                                   |
|      |                           |       |                                   |

# Books I Read This Year

Track the books you have read this school year on the tracking chart below.

| TITLE | AUTHOR | MY THOUGHTS ON THIS BOOK |
|-------|--------|--------------------------|
|       |        |                          |
|       |        |                          |
|       |        |                          |
|       |        |                          |
|       |        |                          |
|       |        |                          |
|       |        |                          |
|       |        |                          |
|       |        |                          |
|       |        |                          |
|       |        |                          |
|       |        |                          |
|       |        |                          |
|       |        |                          |
|       |        |                          |
|       |        |                          |
|       |        |                          |
|       |        |                          |

# Books I Read This Year

Track the books you have read this school year on the tracking chart below.

| TITLE | AUTHOR | MY THOUGHTS ON THIS BOOK |
|-------|--------|--------------------------|
|       |        |                          |
|       |        |                          |
|       |        |                          |
|       |        |                          |
|       |        |                          |
|       |        |                          |
|       |        |                          |
|       |        |                          |
|       |        |                          |
|       |        |                          |
|       |        |                          |
|       |        |                          |
|       |        |                          |
|       |        |                          |
|       |        |                          |
|       |        |                          |
|       |        |                          |
|       |        |                          |
|       |        |                          |

# A Change in Routine

Summertime is coming up! One significant change between being in school and summer break is your routine. While in school, you have a specific routine you follow during the day, at night, and even on weekends. Bedtimes, morning routine, getting to school and class on time, and your after school routine and homework.

Summer can have it's own routine and schedule that can help you do more with your time, help you continue to work on your goals and give you time to continue to make connections and memories with your friends. Use the following activity to help you plan out your summer and make a plan for the next few months.

This summer I am looking forward to _____

_____

This summer I am I worried about _____

_____

This summer, the daily plan is:

| MORNING | |
|---|---|
| AFTERNOON | |
| EVENING | |

**Summer challenge:** Try to challenge yourself to keep practicing what you have learned. Make a list of things you can do this summer to keep practicing your social-emotional learning:

1) _____    2) _____

3) _____    4) _____

5) _____    6) _____

7) _____    8) _____

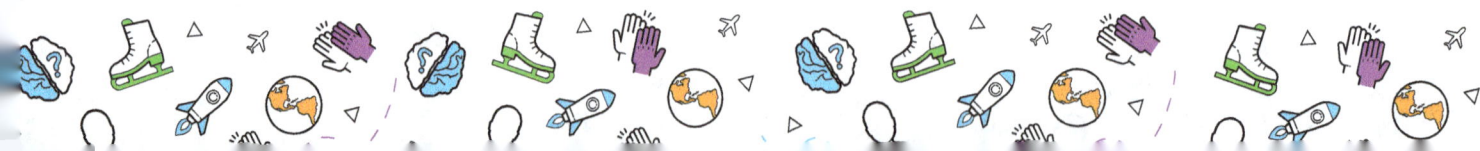

# Read a book this summer!

Here are some can't-put-down summer reads. Use the chart to select the best book for you (and remember you can find these books at your local library, so you don't have to buy the book!).

## FICTION

**Graphic novel** *or* **Inspirational?**

An action-packed Wild West novel!

Read: *Rapunzel's Revenge* by Shannon Hale & Dean Hale

A book about a runaway that will make you laugh and cry.

Read: *Elijah of Buxton* by Christopher Paul Curtis

## NON-FICTION

**Classic** *or* **Sports?**

Cartoons, text and images come together to tell the story of Charlotte Brontë.

Read: *Charlotte Brontë Before Jane Eyre* by Glynnis Fawkes

Basketball and life lessons.

Read: *The Playbook* by Kwame Alexander

Love to read?

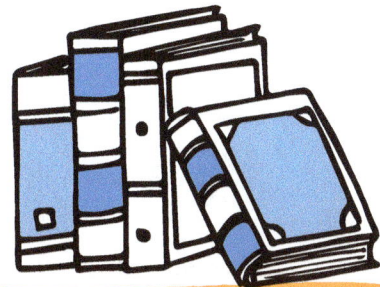

Read all four books! You can find more recommendations from your Librarianor on readbrighty.com

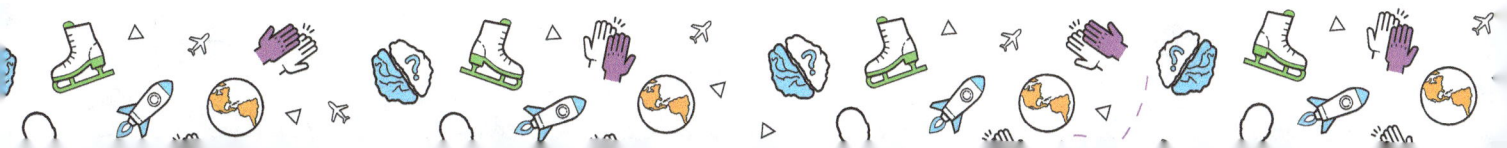

# Social-Emotional Learning Stories

Read the stories below and notice how other students found solutions to their problems using social-emotional learning tools.

## Hollis' story

Hollis loved his art class. He enjoyed expressing himself using color and different materials, and using his hands to create something instead of sitting in class was just plain FUN! Hollis' art teacher was also important to him because she always found a way to encourage him without praising him so much in front of his peers that it became embarrassing. Well, one day, his teacher took one of his paintings that he was working on and held it up in front of the class and professed, "This is a masterpiece! Hollis, this is one of your best works yet, and we must put it on display!" Hollis didn't want the attention and quickly narrowed his eyes and looked straight at the teacher and said: "Just give it back, you're doing too much, and it's not even that good" when he was actually very proud of the hard work he'd done! Why did he respond this way?

If you were Hollis and you were in his position, how would you express yourself?

_____

_____

_____

_____

_____

_____

_____

_____

_____

## Resolution:

In this scenario, Hollis was, in fact, happy for what he'd created, but he allowed for his emotions to overpower his accomplishment. Sometimes, when we're embarrassed about an event or action, we act differently than how we truly feel. When we learn to manage and regulate our emotions, this can be prevented. This can be done by managing your stress and motivating yourself so that way when a situation such as Hollis' arises, you can thoughtfully act, instead of reacting.

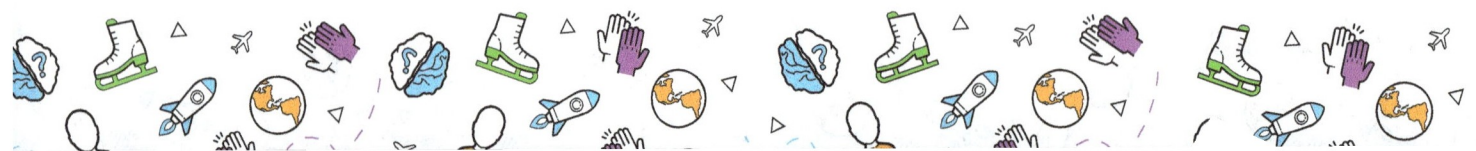

# Social-Emotional Learning Stories

## Jaime's story

Jaime was a perfectionist, and he was unashamed of it. However, because he had to be (and was usually) always right, many of his classmates found him to be arrogant. Jaime's relationships with others became strained because no one wanted to be around him because he would belittle them at any opportunity he got. Jaime didn't mean to do this maliciously, he just had to be right.

How can Jaime learn to allow others to share their opinion without the need to feel dominant?

_____

_____

_____

_____

_____

_____

_____

_____

_____

## Resolution:

Learning how to establish and maintain healthy relationships with your peers and others would help Jaime. Using this social-emotional tool, Jaime could foster better communication and more lasting relationships rather than making others feel small. Although he may mean well, Jaime's actions were very selfish as they were only about his feeling of superiority of others. Jaime needs to learn how to build relationships with others that are fair and mutual. Jaime would need to learn how to be more empathic and work on his listening skills to help him. Being right and feeling like you are the best admittedly feels good; however, it is possible to be the "best" without making others feel small!

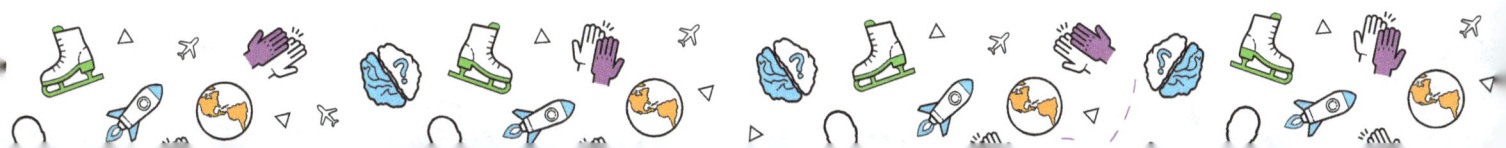

# Self-Care Toolbox

Use this self-care toolbox whenever you need ideas of ways to de-stress or relax. You can write new ideas and share them with your friends, too.

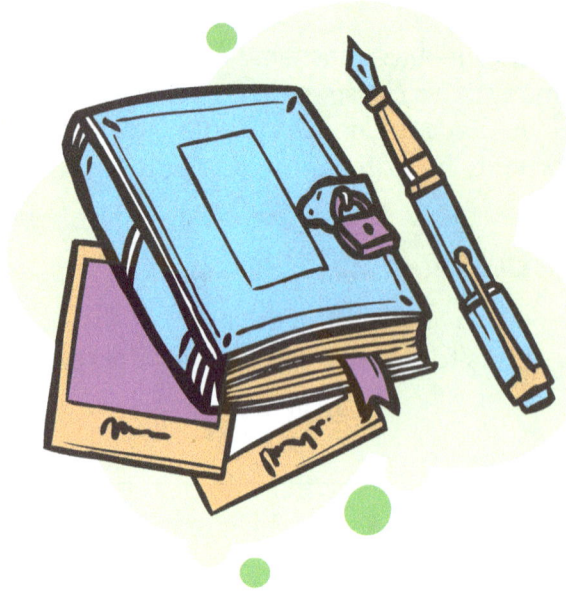

| | | |
|---|---|---|
| Talk to a friend | Journal | Spend quality time with someone |
| Eat a snack | Organize your backpack | Write out your best qualities |
| Go for a bike ride | Play a sport | Share a happy story from childhood |
| Play video games | Read a magazine | Learn how to say hello in another language |
| Listen to music | Stretch your body | Research your dream job |
| Cook | Write a poem | Take an extra long shower |
| Draw | Read about a country you'd like to visit | Get a makeover or haircut |
| Play music | Go shopping | Organize the house |
| Read the news | Make fun plans | Write a short story |
| Take photos of nature | Read a book | Read feel-good quotes |
| Yoga | Take a nap | Learn about college |
| Have a healing chat | Watch a movie or TV show | Lift weights |
| Take a bath | Immerse yourself in nature | Volunteer your time |
| Walk the dog | Play cards or a board game | Commit a random act of kindness |
| Clean your room | Sing | Eat your favorite food |

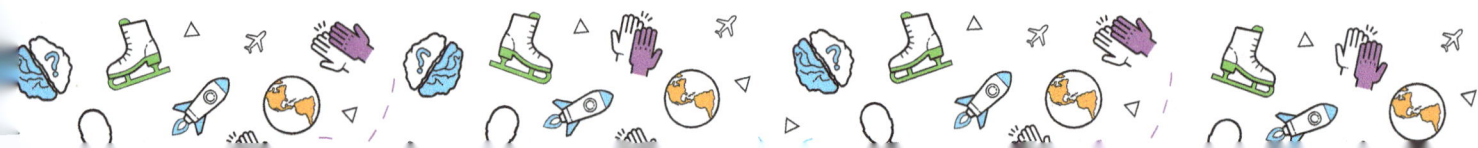

# Mindful Breathing

Use these techniques to calm your body and mind, and breathe mindfully.

## Hot Chocolate Breathing

Imagine you are holding a cup of hot chocolate, and you are blowing the little marshmallows around and cooling off your cup. Take in a deep breath, then exhale through your mouth to blow those tiny marshmallows around your cup. Repeat three to five times.

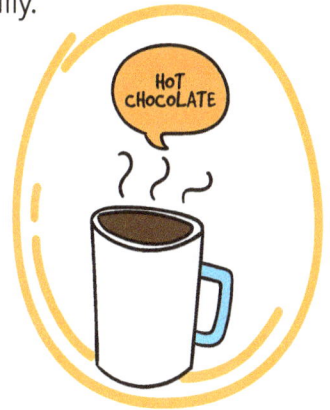

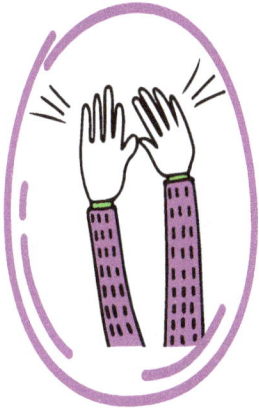

## Hand Tracing Breathing

Use your pencil and trace your hand on this page (It's ok if you mark over the text - you can still read it). Now use your drawing to breathe in and out as you trace your fingers around your hand. Start below your thumb and as you trace the line up your thumb, breathe in, and as you trace your thumb down toward your finger, breathe out. Breathe in and out slowly as you trace up and down your fingers.

## Flower Breathing

Imagine you are holding a flower, maybe a dandelion that is soft and puffy white. Take in a deep breath, then exhale through your mouth to blow those fluffy white puffs into the air. Repeat three to five times to blow all of the puffs off of the stem.

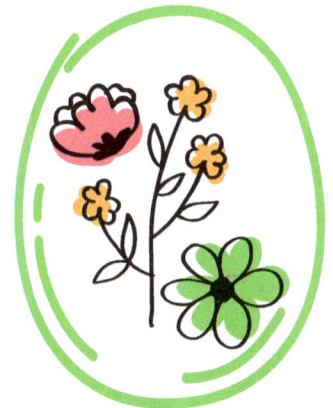

## Counting to 10

First, sit with your feet on the floor and close your eyes. Count to 10 for each breath in this way:

Breathe in = 1
Breathe out = 2
Breathe in = 3
Breathe out = 4
Breathe in = 5
Breathe out = 6
Breathe in = 7
Breathe out = 8
Breathe in = 9
Breathe out = 10

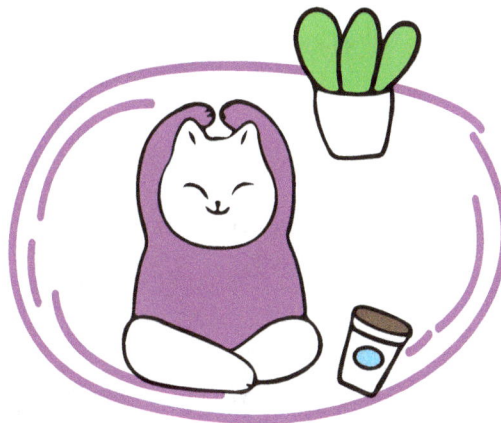

Then, start over. If you find that you've lost focus and are at number 12, start back at one again.

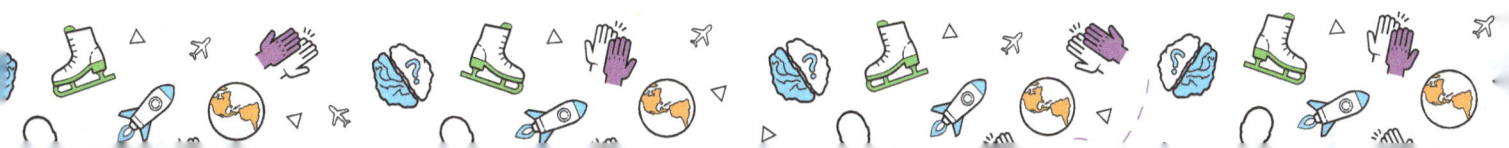

# Countdown to Calm

Use this 5-step countdown whenever you need to calm down from an upsetting situation. Whatever you do, remember that calming down is the best way to prevent things from getting worse, so just lean on these tips whenever you need to feel better after or during a tough moment.

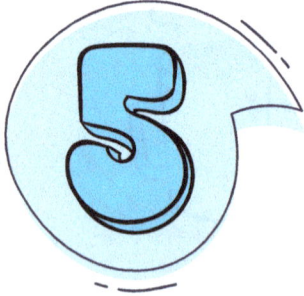

### 5 Minutes to walk away from whatever or whoever has you feeling upset

*Removing yourself from an argument or task that has frustrated you is the first step to feeling calm. Go for a quick walk, ask to step into the hallway, or go to the bathroom and splash some cold water on your face.*

### 4 Emotions you can name you are experiencing

*Naming your emotions will help you regain clarity. It is easy to feel overwhelmed when you're angry or upset, so identifying exactly how you are feeling will help you communicate to others exactly what is going on inside of you.*

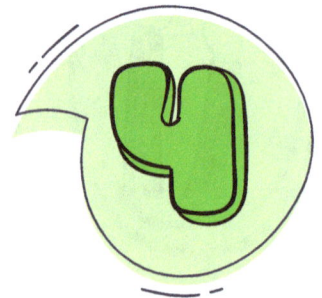

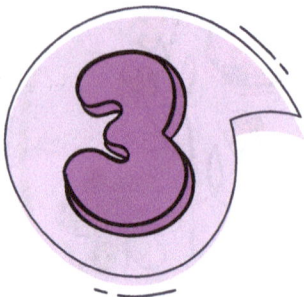

### 3 Things you need to communicate

*What is it that you want and need to say now to help heal the situation or move forward? Write or mentally store three things you need to communicate with others to express your needs. Be sure to be brave and honest!*

### 2 Actions you can take

*What are TWO specific things you can do to bring about a solution? These could be things you do, say, or a person you bring into the conversation.*

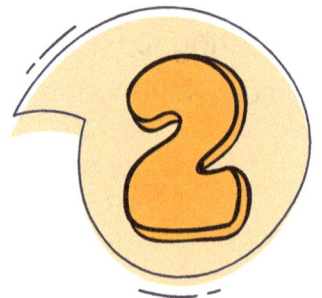

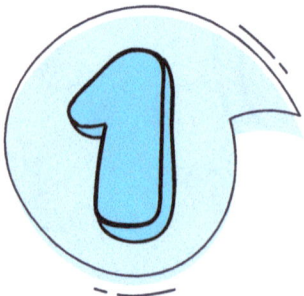

### 1 Person you can go to for support

*Who is there right now, or who can you identify that can lend their support to you? Do you need an adult to come in and help fix a fight? Or do you need help studying to do better on a test the next time? Knowing and naming who you are going to go to for ongoing help will make you more likely to reach out.*

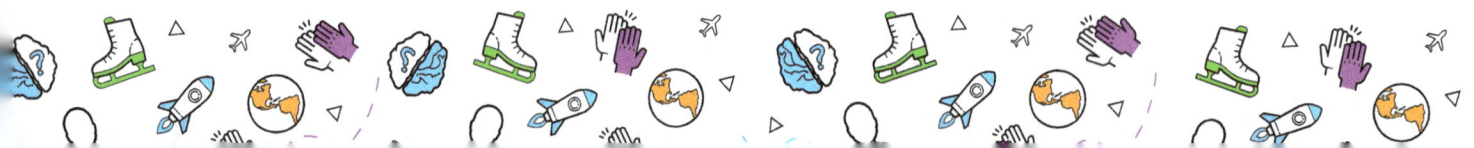

# Top 10 Habits of Social Emotional Learning

**1.** Journal to reflect upon my emotions, thoughts, and experiences.

**2.** Practice a growth mindset through replacing fixed thoughts.

**3.** Set intentions for my day or a class.

**4.** Talk with people from different places or different perspectives.

**5.** Resolve conflicts peacefully and disagree respectfully.

**6.** Utilize positive coping skills to manage stress.

**7.** Make good decisions that keep others and me safe.

**8.** Create and accomplish positive goals.

**9.** Ask for help from a trusted adult when I need it.

**10.** Practice kindness to others and myself.

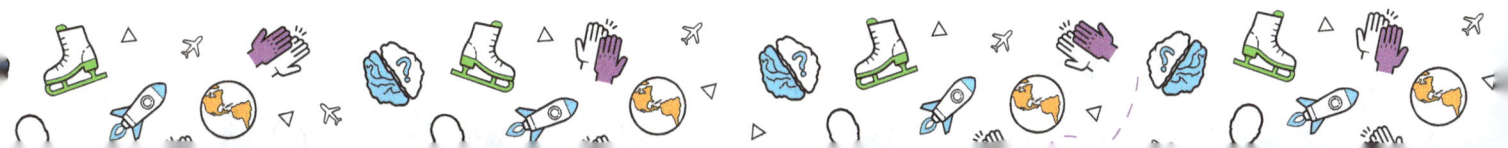

# Social-Emotional Learning Skills Checklist

Place a checkmark next to the skills in which you feel you are strong. Leave the box blank if you need additional help in practicing that skill.

- ◯ I can identify and name my emotions.

- ◯ I can ask for help when I need it (both at school and personally)

- ◯ I can identify and name what I am good at

- ◯ I am confident in my abilities.

- ◯ Even when things seem too difficult, I try and think I can succeed with hard work.

- ◯ I can manage stress by making healthy choices.

- ◯ I can motivate myself, even when I feel discouraged.

- ◯ I can set goals for myself and achieve them.

- ◯ I control my emotions so I don't make choices that harm myself or others, or that I regret.

- ◯ I can understand things by placing myself in someone else's shoes.

- ◯ I accept and respect that people have a variety of experiences and perspectives.

- ◯ I can explain the value of diversity and how it enriches environments.

- ◯ I can communicate my needs clearly and appropriately.

- ◯ I am a good listener.

- ◯ I can work well in teams and am willing to cooperate and compromise.

- ◯ I feel confident in who I am and can stand up to social pressures.

- ◯ I make safe, appropriate, and ethical choices that do not bring harm to others nor myself.

- ◯ I work to identify problems and form constructive solutions both in and outside of school.

- ◯ I engage in self-reflection to make decisions that positively impact my physical, emotional, and mental health.

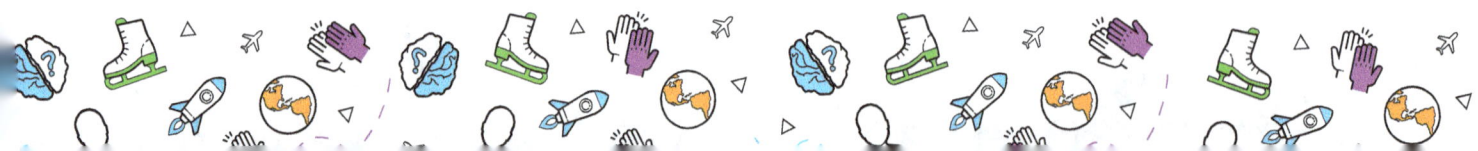

# Self-Talk Affirmations

Affirmations are encouraging sentences. We can say these encouragements to ourselves to help us have a positive mindset and feel better about ourselves.

I love myself.

I can be flexible.

I am bold.

I can get better.

I am brave.

I am thankful.

I am strong.

It is OK to make mistakes.

I can try new things.

I am a mathematician.

I am a scientist.

I am a writer.

I am adventurous.

I can do this.

I can persevere.

I can calm myself down.

I can listen carefully.

I can ask for help.

I can take charge.

I am enough.

I get better every single day.

I am an amazing person.

All of my problems have solutions.

Today I am a leader.

I forgive myself for my mistakes.

My challenges help me grow.

My mistakes help me learn and grow.

I have courage and confidence.

I can control my own happiness.

I can make a difference.

Today I choose to be confident.

I am kind.

I am special.

I am loved.

I am a reader.

I can say no.

I can help.

I can control my own happiness.

My positive thoughts create positive feelings.

Every day is a fresh start.

I can get through anything.

Today I choose to think positively.

It's okay not to know everything.

I believe in my goals and dreams.

I can do anything I put my mind to.

If I fall, I will get back up again.

It is enough to do my best.

I am capable of so much.

I have what I need for right now.

I can do better next time.

I believe in myself.

Today is going to be awesome.

I only compare myself to myself.

I am a good friend.

I can make a difference.

I believe in myself and my abilities

I can be a leader.

I matter.

I will be OK.

It is OK to feel this way.

I have something to say.

I can resolve this conflict.

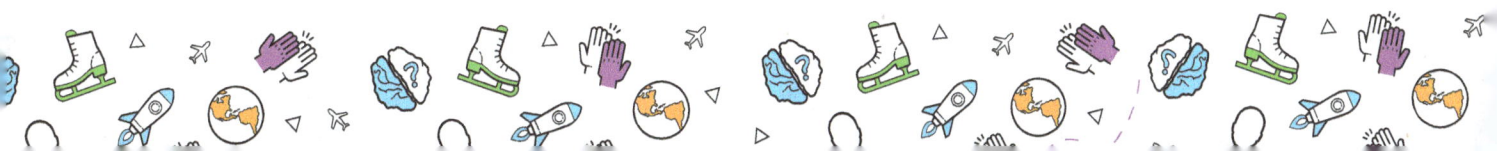

All the Planners in the series:

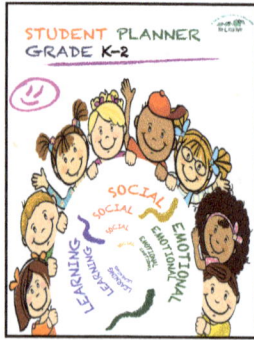

Social Emotional Learning
(SEL) Student Planner
Grades K-2
ISBN: 978-1-7336417-0-8

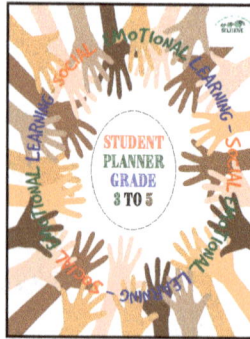

Social Emotional Learning
(SEL) Student Planner
Grades 3-5
ISBN: 978-1-7336417-1-5

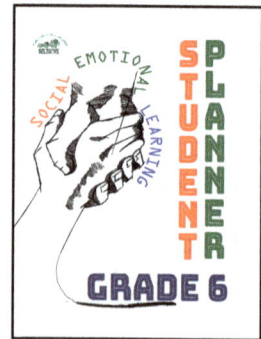

Social Emotional Learning
(SEL) Student Planner
Grade 6
ISBN: 978-1-7336417-2-2

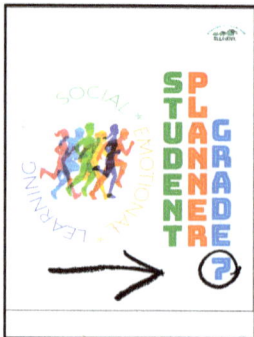

Social Emotional Learning
(SEL) Student Planner
Grade 7
ISBN: 978-1-7336417-3-9

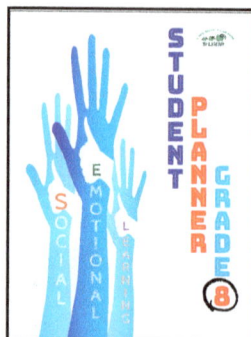

Social Emotional Learning
(SEL) Student Planner
Grade 8
ISBN: 978-1-7336417-7-7

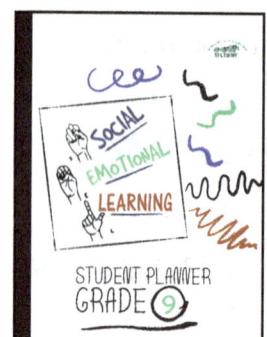

Social Emotional Learning
(SEL) Student Planner
Grade 9
ISBN: 978-1-7336417-8-4

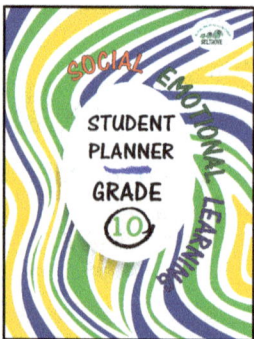

Social Emotional Learning
(SEL) Student Planner
Grade 10
ISBN: 978-1-7336417-9-1

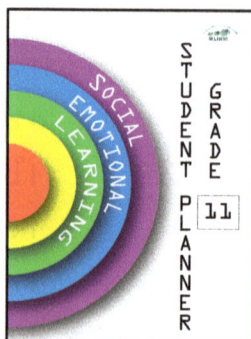

Social Emotional Learning
(SEL) Student Planner
Grade 11
ISBN: 978-1-7336417-4-6

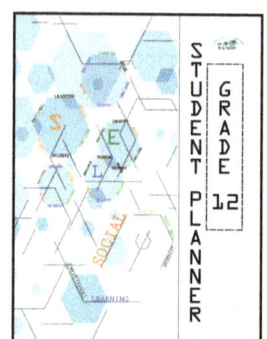

Social Emotional Learning
(SEL) Student Planner
Grade 12
ISBN: 978-1-7336417-5-3

For further information go to www.seltrove.com